FINDING THE GOOD

A SELF-CARE WORKBOOK FOR CAREGIVERS

Carol Chapman

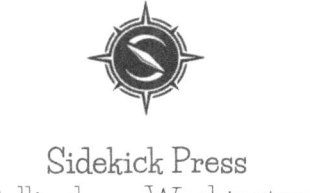

Sidekick Press
Bellingham, Washington

Publisher's Note:
This book details the author's personal experiences with and opinions about health and happiness. The author is not a doctor/physician, nurse, physician's assistant, advanced practice nurse, psychiatrist, psychologist, therapist, counselor, social worker, or any other medical or mental health provider. The author and publisher are providing this book and its contents on an "as is" basis and make no representations or warranties of any kind with respect to this book or its contents. The author and publisher disclaim all such representations and warranties, including, for example, warranties of merchantability and health care for a particular purpose. In addition, the author and publisher do not represent or warrant that the information accessible via this book is accurate, complete, or current. Statements made in this book are not intended to diagnose, treat, cure, or prevent any condition or disease. Please consult with your own physician or health care specialist regarding the suggestions and recommendations made in this book. Except as specifically stated in this book, neither the author nor publisher, nor any authors, contributors, nor other representatives will be liable for damages arising out of or in connection with the use of this book. This is a comprehensive limitation of liability that applies to all damages of any kind, including (without limitation) compensatory; direct, indirect, or consequential damages; loss of data, income, or profit; loss of or damage to property and claims of third parties. You understand that this book is not intended as a substitute for consultation with licensed professionals. This book provides content related to physical and/or mental health issues. As such, use of this book implies your acceptance of this disclaimer.

Published 2025
Printed in the United States of America
ISBN: 978-1-958808-45-0

Sidekick Press
2950 Newmarket Street, Suite 101-329
Bellingham, Washington 98226
sidekickpress.com

Finding the Good: A Self-Care Workbook for Caregivers

Cover design by Andrea Gabriel

Also by Carol Chapman:
Finding the Good: A Journey through Love, Loss, and Living

Carol lives with her favorite guy, Barney Pembroke Welsh Corgi Chapman, in her native state of Wyoming. Read more about Carol and finding the good in everyday life at https://carolchapmanwrites.com.

Contents

INTRODUCTION

How This Book Can Help You

Stop! Take a breath.

Admitting you're scared when your loved one experiences a health crisis doesn't make you weak—it makes you honest.

After all, this is a frightening moment. One minute, your life was moving along as usual. The next, everything changed. Suddenly, you've been pulled into a world of medical decisions, uncertainty, and nonstop responsibility. Tasks you may have never handled before—finances, appointments, medications, meals—are now entirely on your shoulders. You're grieving the life you had while trying to hold together the one unfolding in front of you.

You will get through this. I did. But not without the guidance and support of others. That's why I'm here for you now.

When my husband experienced an unexpected seizure that led to a prolonged health battle, I too was unprepared. In a matter of hours, everything shifted. The fear and overwhelm were constant, but so was the love. That love kept me going, even when I had nothing left to give.

This workbook follows my memoir, *Finding the Good: A Journey of Love, Loss, and Living* (2024), which details the emotional, physical, and spiritual challenges of caregiving. By sharing my experiences—including the things I learned the hard way—I hope to make your journey a little easier. This workbook is filled with tools, reflections, and gentle guidance to help you care not only for your loved one but for yourself. Because your needs matter. Your health matters. And, you are not alone.

I'm not a grief counselor, a psychiatrist, a doctor, or a minister. However, I possess unique qualifications for writing this book that others may lack. I have been in the trenches. I was a caregiver who watched for two-and-a-half years while my beloved husband slowly lost himself to an uncontrollable growth in the center of his brain. I experienced the pain and frustration of not being able to do anything but be with him and help him during his slow walk toward death.

For those two-and-a-half years, our life circled around his illness, and I spent long hours by his bedside. Our positive attitudes wavered as we faced the roller coaster of life with a terminal illness. Stress—there was always stress.

As the primary caregiver with no instruction book and no idea how to navigate taking care of the man I was still crazy about, I searched for common sense tips to help me through this horrifying situation.

How was I supposed to feel? How did others cope with being tossed into the confusing and terrifying ocean of traumatic or terminal illness? Larry was in a huge hospital in a city unfamiliar to both of us. Trial and error became my teacher. I learned I was stronger and more capable than I'd realized.

One of my key lessons? You, as a caregiver, must take care of your own health, both mentally and physically. If you fall sick, who will take your place as the caregiver? Self-care is a commitment that includes managing emotions, as well as learning how to be your loved one's advocate.

Becoming a good caregiver is a process. In caring for my husband, I made mistakes and had to learn from those mistakes—sometimes in uncomfortable ways—before I found a way to adjust. As you travel this path, try to learn from any errors you make, and be forgiving and gentle with yourself as you do.

Keep in mind that not everything in this book will resonate exactly with your caregiving experiences. My husband was battling cancer, for instance, a disease with common features and caregiving responsibilities but its own unique path. What worked for me might not be right for you. People don't all react the same in similar situations, and your feelings may not mirror mine. But the principles of supporting a loved one struggling through illness while caring for oneself are universal: no one benefits by managing this journey alone. This workbook is there for you, regardless of your circumstances—the caregiving manual I wish I could have consulted myself.

The focus of the first part of the book is on self-care and its many repercussions. I've suggested ideas and options for your consideration. You might find it helpful to use a colored marker or a pen to highlight the tips and suggestions most beneficial to you. Locating them later will be quicker that way.

You're also sure to benefit from taking the time to fill out the included worksheets. The process of writing things down—rather than just reading and moving on—will allow you to delve deeper into your experiences and find the best ways to address whatever problems arise.

The second portion of the book contains simple activities and art projects for you to pursue during idle times. When your hands are busy, your mind is distracted from that constant worry you may be feeling. You'll find directions and patterns for how to benefit from these activities. These ideas are designed to bolster your attitude throughout this challenging journey. Please try them out for stress relief.

Now take another deep, soothing breath, and read on . . .

ONE

Our Story

Larry, my college sweetheart and husband of thirty-eight years, and I had sold our small trucking company and decided to take a vacation driving from our home in Casper, Wyoming, to Anchorage, Alaska. Riding in our motor home with our dogs, Hector Welsh Corgi and Ollie Sheltie, we enjoyed the first days of our trip.

On day five, Larry complained of a headache he couldn't shake. He often took over-the-counter headache pills, and he had a prescription for migraine medicine from our family doctor. We both believed he just needed more time to let the drugs work.

The next day, after we crossed the border from Canada into Alaska, the first town we came to was Tok. As we drove toward our campground, I noticed an InstaCare building. Little did I know we'd soon be speeding toward it.

Larry hadn't been acting like his normal self. After he parked our RV in our reserved space, he continued to sit in the driver's seat instead of getting out to level the rig and hook up the utilities.

Something is wrong with him. A doctor needs to see him right away.

I raced the two of us to the InstaCare I'd seen earlier, and a nurse and doctor helped Larry into the clinic where he had two subsequent seizures. The doctor couldn't do anything for him except arrange to fly us to Providence Hospital in Anchorage, nearly 300 miles away.

The next morning, a stern-looking neuro-oncologist diagnosed Larry with the deadliest brain tumor a person can get—a glioblastoma multiforme tumor located in the communication center of his brain.

Surely that couldn't be right! He'd been okay eighteen hours earlier.

Larry was now lying there before me, unresponsive. Suddenly, I had so many decisions to make. Without children or living parents, I became responsible for things I felt unequipped to handle. I'd never made serious decisions like this on my own. Never!

"We can start treatment here right away," the neuro-oncologist said. "But if you don't want him to have it here, you need to decide what you want to do. This is a very aggressive cancer. Time is important."

I felt confused and overwhelmed. A decision had to be made about treatment. Our two dogs were still in the RV in Tok. My mind couldn't think in a logical manner. I was jittery and I still didn't know what to do.

Having done a lot of truck dispatching for our company, I asked the nurse for a pad of paper and a pen. I began writing the things that were of immediate concern.

1. Where should Larry have treatment?

2. What about our dogs?

3. How do I get our RV and the dark green Chevy pickup returned to Casper?

Making this list gave me something to focus my thoughts on, and it occupied my hands. As I made notes, my heart slowed, and I became calmer.

Starting with number one, using the information I had, I made the best decision I could make at the time. Larry would get treatment in Denver, Colorado, which was slightly less than 300 miles from our home in Casper. Our nephew had seen a neuro-oncologist who treated his brain tumor at Swedish Hospital in Englewood, a Denver suburb.

Once I decided on the treatment location, the Anchorage hospital social worker took over the logistics of arranging transportation, notifying the doctor and hospital, and other details.

Now that the first question of where Larry would receive treatment was checked off my list, it was easier to arrange for the dogs and RV to be transported home.

I would become Larry's primary caregiver. During the next two-and-a-half years, we would live mainly in our RV in Englewood. With a space at the Flying Saucer Campground, we would be less than ten minutes from help at Swedish Hospital.

As I had to learn the hard way, the devastating news of a sudden illness or accident can knock you for a loop. It's difficult to think clearly. After the initial shock wore off, however, organizing what needed to be done immediately helped get me moving. A list of the top three most pressing decisions grounded me. I regained a small amount of control, which helped me move on to whatever came next. There had to be a beginning plan . . . a place to start. By putting pen to paper, I found one.

TWO

Making Decisions

When your loved one falls ill or receives an unexpected diagnosis, you may be the only one making decisions about his or her care, including where to get the necessary medical help. If your loved one is able to give input, discuss the choices best for both of you. Otherwise, if someone you trust is available, especially someone who has faced similar circumstances, listen to that person's advice. That doesn't mean always doing what they suggest but listening to what they have to say. Consider your position and your options. Now is the time to announce what you want, including what is most convenient for you and your family.

Remember that you will be able to adjust most plans that turn out to be unworkable, but you need to think of what's most important in the moment.

Once you've made those first few decisions, don't spend your time worrying about them. You'll have other important things to consider. If people grumble, remember it isn't their life to live—it's yours. Keep in mind that you know yourself and the patient better than others do.

Do the best you can. Your situation may be long term. It's inevitable that circumstances will change in the upcoming days and weeks, and you'll have other decisions to make.

Trust yourself, first and foremost, and give yourself credit for tackling these difficult decisions on your own.

WORKSHEET - WHAT ARE YOUR FIRST THREE MAJOR DECISIONS?

You've just been hit by the lightning bolt of a loved one's illness. Take a few deep breaths to calm yourself. List the three most important decisions you need to make. By writing them down, your feeling of loss of control will ease. Know that you've already been able to make some key decisions about the future.

1.
2.
3.

WORKSHEET - CHOOSING A DOCTOR

In considering care for your loved one, ask yourself: would you rather go to the doctor who sees the condition *once in six months* or the doctor who deals with it *every day*?

You likely won't know the answer to this question right now. That's okay. Work your way through the process. Move as quickly as possible.

Before you start your search, answer the following:

- What is the diagnosis?

- What type of doctor is needed?

- Which doctors are in your area?

- Are you able to go to another city for the best treatment if necessary?

- Is the doctor affiliated with a hospital you prefer?

- Are the doctor and hospital covered by your insurance (and if you are in the U.S., are they on your company's approved list)?

How to find the best doctor:

- Talk to your patient's primary physician.

- Ask the insurance agent if he or she is familiar with a specialist in your area.

- Talk to someone who has faced a similar situation.

- Consult family and friends.

- Contact a crisis center.

- Do an online search for recommended specialists.

An online search will give you information on the doctor's board certification, specialty training, hospital affiliation, etc. In some cases, your choice of doctor and/or hospital may be limited, especially if you live in a rural area. There may not be another qualified doctor nearby. Then, you'll need to accept the available specialist or plan to travel to another location.

Meet with the doctor as soon as possible. Take some notes at your initial meeting:
Was the doctor on time for his or her appointment?
How did the doctor treat you? Do you like him or her?
Did he or she listen to you or show signs of not paying attention?
Did you feel a level of trust with the doctor?
Did the doctor's staff seem supportive?

If the first doctor doesn't fit for some reason and you want to interview a different one, here is a second worksheet.

Was the doctor on time for his or her appointment?
How did the doctor treat you? Do you like him or her?
Did he or she listen to you or show signs of not paying attention?
Did you feel a level of trust with the doctor?
Did the doctor's staff seem supportive?

Factors to consider for treatment:
Distance of the treatment center from your home?
Will treatment require travel and being away overnight? If so, where will you stay?
Who will care for your home, animals, and children if treatment requires you to be away from them?

Other considerations:
Will treatment require hospital stays?
Are there limitations to your loved one's mobility?
Will your loved one need twenty-four-hour care?

Now that you've evaluated all of the factors involved in your loved one's treatment, you've made some of the hardest decisions yet. Good job!

THREE

Dealing with the Medical Profession

Early on in Larry's illness, I found myself in conflict with a doctor over Larry's care. Larry had spent three weeks in the hospital—with two of those in the rehab area—and had become depressed. I felt he should go home, while the doctor wanted him to stay longer in the hospital. I spoke up, because I believed I knew Larry's mental condition. The doctor oversaw a wing full of patients and only saw numbers on a chart. I was with Larry every day; it was my job to advocate for him.

As difficult as it is, you may find yourself in similar circumstances: standing up to a professional because you know what's best. I encourage you to challenge the doctor as needed, particularly when it comes to the personal needs of your loved one—concerns the doctor doesn't always know or understand.

You are the voice for your ailing loved one. You must represent what's best when someone can't speak for themselves. Some things to keep in mind:

- Your loved one is not a number on a chart! He or she is much more than that and must be treated accordingly. Generally, doctors realize you know the patient better than they do, and they will listen to what you say. If not, you'll need to trust your intuition and speak against the doctor's wishes as necessary.

- If you feel a professional is being harsh or bullying the patient, step in and tell that person he or she has pushed far enough.

- Don't be cowed by a doctor if you feel his or her decision isn't right. Ask for an explanation.

- Sometimes a nurse will intervene when a doctor's orders don't seem right. When that doesn't happen, you may be the one who needs to intercede.

- As an advocate, it's your job to see that one doctor works with the other doctors. For example, in the absence of the main doctor in charge of your loved one's case, a doctor on temporary assignment, such as one working in a skilled nursing facility, may try to change your loved one's prescribed medication. You need to know which doctor has the final say about your loved one's care.

- When multiple doctors are involved, including a primary doctor, hospital doctors, and specialists, it's important that the primary doctor be kept informed. All hospital and specialist records should be sent to the primary doctor or that doctor can't be of much help. When your loved one has an appointment with the primary doctor, ask if that doctor has seen all the necessary reports.

- If your loved one is in the hospital, try to find out when the doctor makes the rounds so you can be there in person. A nurse may be able to relay this information or give you an idea of what the doctor said in your absence. But whenever possible, time your visits to coincide with the doctor's. They don't make their schedules to fit yours, so you'll have to try to fit theirs.

- Appointments, tests, and treatments don't always run on the planned schedule. Be prepared to wait or be flexible. And if you are a few minutes late for an appointment and you have a legitimate reason for doing so, maintain good relations with your loved one's medical professionals by explaining why the patient is late.

Always try to make friends with the nurses and certified nursing assistants (CNAs) at the hospital and doctor's office. They work incredibly hard and are invaluable for your piece of mind (as well as being helpful sources of information). When you aren't there, you'll feel more comfortable knowing who's going to be watching out for your loved one.

Don't forget to thank them with words and in other simple ways.

1. If your patient receives too many flowers, take a vase or two to the nurses' station for them to enjoy.

2. You have no obligation to give gifts to hospital or doctor's office employees, but nurses, CNAs, and other professional workers love chocolate. If you do bring a treat, don't forget the person who cleans the room.

3. Even though the situation may be grim, try to put a smile on your face during appointments. A smile costs so little and bolsters others while it helps you feel happier.

4. Your loved one may receive better care from hospital or clinic staff if they know you often spend time with their patient or tend to pop in at unscheduled times.

While I'm on the subject of medical care, here are a few words about pharmacists—another essential person in the chain of help surrounding you.

1. If your normal pharmacy can't fill at least a partial prescription order, ask them to call around to other pharmacies in the area. Someone will likely carry enough medicine to fill the gap until your order can be filled.

2. In my experience, I usually couldn't get an entire prescription order filled the first time I went to the pharmacy with a new prescription or even a refill. It often took two trips to the pharmacy to get the full amount. If this happens to you, remember it doesn't do you or the pharmacist any good to get angry about it. Just do what you have to do and move on.

3. When you pick up refilled prescriptions, check to see if the pills or liquids appear to look like the previous medication. If the color, size, or shape is different, ask the pharmacist about it. Although your order may look unusual, the pharmacy may have ordered from another company. It's your job to check and make sure.

4. Unless your doctor has approved it, don't let a pharmacist help you by recommending a generic brand. Depending on the type of drug that's prescribed, the generic brand may not offer exactly the same benefits. I found that out when a pharmacist recommended that I switch to a generic brand for Larry's anti-seizure drug. In the end, the switch didn't make any difference in Larry's case, but it taught me a valuable lesson for future reference.

5. Mail-order prescriptions can present challenges, because the drugs may face delays in shipping. Some insurance plans require policyholders to use this type of pharmacy, so be sure to order these prescriptions well in advance. In the U.S., your insurance company will need to handle any payment issues, but you might need to pay up front to initiate shipping.

6. If an order arrives in unsatisfactory condition, call and request to speak to the manager rather than the receptionist or whoever answers the phone. Explain the situation and how urgent the drug is to the patient. As a last resort, ask a nurse from your doctor's office to contact the mail-order pharmacy. They can get results, even if you can't.

Sometimes it can seem like there are more issues for a caregiver than you might be able to handle. Take a deep breath, stand up straight, and do your best. You can't do more than that—and you're already doing a great job just by being there.

FOUR

Things You Are Going to Need Now

Once you have a diagnosis and a plan of action for your loved one, the first thing to arm yourself with is a way of keeping track of everything the doctor tells you and the patient. Our retention of what we hear is often forgotten before we reach the parking lot.

Purchase a notebook to carry with you to all appointments. Although some people are able to keep all this information on their smartphone, I would have found it impossible to quickly locate pertinent data while I hunted for it in my phone.

Things you'll need:

- A notebook or other place to keep track of the following:
    - Medicine changes
    - New drugs
    - Eliminated drugs
    - Dosages and any dosage changes
    - Directions or comments from the doctor
- To manage appointments, add a small calendar to your notebook to keep track and avoid over-booking.
- Observe and take note of changes in your loved one's appetite, energy level, mood, or basic bodily functions.
- If questions arise, jot them down as you think of them.
- Remember to ask for the spellings of medications or terms you don't know—you may need to refer to these in your roles as patient-advocate and caregiver.

FIVE

Paperwork You May Need Later

For those of us who rely on private insurance to manage our loved one's care: your life will be easier later if you designate a storage box or bin for keeping your documents in case of insurance denials and for income tax reports. Even if you simply toss these materials in, it's much easier to find items when they're gathered in one place.

Things to keep:

- Medical records and reports

- Correspondence pertaining to the patient

- Receipts for medical supplies and purchased or rental equipment

- Health insurance premium payments

- Copies of benefits paid by insurances

- Medicare and secondary insurance premium payments

- Any fundraiser income and expenses (if you paid for them)

- Any income you receive

- Travel receipts for medical treatments

Your tax preparer will know which of the items can be applied to your individual return. They may advise you to keep all paperwork for a period of seven years. You don't know what may be needed. Later you can throw out the unnecessary pages.

WORKSHEET — SPECIAL EQUIPMENT

As caregiver, ask yourself which pieces of special equipment you will need for your loved one:

	Hospital bed
	Toilet lifter
	Portable toilet
	Shower stool
	Handlebars for the shower, bathtub, and/or stairs
	Crutches
	Walker
	Cane
	Wheelchair
	Home oxygen
	Humidifier
	Sheet protectors or pads
	Other equipment as required

You can obtain these items as rentals, loans, or purchases from a variety of places. Check with the hospital or caregiving facility, or look online for supplier suggestions. Rentals or loans can be worthwhile options, especially since your loved one's special equipment needs will likely change over time.

SIX

You May Have To Do It All Now

Part of the reason primary caregivers suffer from burnout is because they must suddenly do the job of two people—including all the day-to-day upkeep for a home, vehicles, and other necessary items. Before your loved one became ill, it might have been easy to overlook the things he or she did to ease your burdens. You didn't have to take care of everything by yourself. Now, all of those expectations may be on you.

A task like making coffee each night before going to bed might be one of the simple things your partner did. It's easy to take acts like these for granted. Then, one day, your loved one can't do even modest chores. Suddenly, it's your obligation to have the coffee ready, manage the child and pet care, the vehicle and house needs, and dozens of other things you'd never thought about because you had a helpful companion. Now, here you are. You have to do it all—on top of your role as advocate and caregiver.

In addition to managing your home life, you may also be responsible for arranging and ferrying your loved one to and from all appointments. If you have children, you'll be tending to them too: their needs aren't going to disappear just because your loved one is ill.

If the ill person is an aging parent, you'll have responsibilities like paying their bills, arranging and going to doctor appointments, managing their medications, and many other tasks.

Do you have a job? What about it? How is that going to work?

Your new responsibilities can easily overwhelm you. When adding in the stress of not knowing what kind of future you will face, it's no wonder you're exhausted by the end of the day!

With the new burdens you're facing, you may feel resentful, even though you know your loved one didn't ask for the illness or accident. It happened! With it came the additional roles you are required to take on—roles that only increases your stress level.

Whenever Larry and I planned the nearly 300-mile trip home to Casper from the Flying Saucer Campground in Englewood, it became my responsibility to decide what day we'd go—depending on his treatment schedule and allowing for a couple of rest days afterward. I'd gather up the laundry, pack what few clothes we'd need, and arrange the medications, making sure refills wouldn't be required while we were gone. I'd organize the dogs' toys and food, blankets, snacks, several bottles of water, and whatever else I thought we might need while we traveled.

Sadly, I'd become irritated because, while I made numerous trips from the RV to the vehicle, Larry sat in his favorite recliner and watched me climb down the steps of the RV with my arms loaded. After I'd piled those items on the back seat of the pickup, left room for the dogs, and climbed back into the RV, he'd still be sitting right in the same place. *I have to do it all!*

He wasn't immune to my concerns. He'd often say, "I wish I could help do that." But the reality was, he didn't have the strength to do any of these tasks.

Even while Larry felt distressed to see me doing everything—and the situation wasn't his fault—irritation gnawed at me. *Maybe he'll be strong enough to help next time*, I'd think. But I knew that wasn't going to happen. In the meantime, I had to learn to manage my frustration.

The buildup of stress for primary caregivers frequently causes anger and irritation. To avoid lashing out—or getting ill or injured yourself—it's important to tackle this problem.

To help lower the pressure, try these three things:

1. Get organized (lists, lists, lists).

2. Set your priorities.

3. Delegate tasks and ask for help when you need it.

Is making lists and setting priorities and delegating going to solve all of your stress problems? Absolutely not. But focusing on what you can do (or even intend to do) may provide some relief, and it could possibly return a small sense of control to you.

Consider the following:

- Most people want to help, but they don't know what to do. Delegate those tasks you'd like someone else to handle. Can your brother or dad take the car for an oil change? Will your friend pick up milk and eggs so you don't need to go to the store? Can your cousin come sit with your loved one for an hour or so to give you a chance to get out?

- If your family isn't able to assist you and, even if they are, think of friends who might have free time and be available. Some church groups or fellow workers are awesome at doing chores you can't do yourself. Don't forget about teenagers and neighbors.

- It's difficult to ask others for help, but this is a time when you can't do it all. Any forms of aid will give you a better sense of security. This management of your life by committee is going to be your reality for a while, so make it as easy on yourself as you can.

- Keep in mind that other people, even family members, have their own busy lives. While you are uppermost in their thoughts at the beginning of a tragic illness or accident, their routines and activities may lure them away. It's not that they don't care. They have their own concerns. Try not to be hurt if your friends from work stop calling as frequently. You're stuck in your situation. They aren't.

- Strangers may offer to help but be leery of anyone offering to bring you cheaper medications from a foreign country. Consult your doctor before you agree to anything like this. Even though someone says they know of a treatment for an illness because "their sister had the exact same thing," again, talk it over with your doctor first.

Lastly, try to make the most of tasks that offer moments of relief. I dreaded driving, but when the dogs and Larry were loaded in the pickup, and we started down the highway with the radio playing, I'd feel better. I was getting things done.

You are doing so well. Keep moving forward. You can do this!

WORKSHEET - THINGS YOU NEED HELP WITH NOW

When you're a caregiver seeking aid from family, friends, or a professional service, you'll find it easier to make a list of the things you need help with. After you've identified those things, find someone who can help you. The sample worksheet, below. allows you to keep track of the necessary tasks and who will help with each one.

Task	Who Can Help

WORKSHEET - FINDING HELP

Your worksheet will tell you what kind of help you need, and then you'll need to figure out how to find those helpers. Here's a list of resources.

Which of these people or organizations have you contacted? Put a check beside each of them.

	Ask friends and family for ideas of the various service providers they already know about.
	If you belong to a church, ask your pastor or church secretary to suggest volunteers to do chores for you.
	Remember that teenage neighbors are often available and even eager to help.
	Look online for reputable or bonded/licensed health services. Compare their costs and services.
	Call your city human resources division and ask if they can recommend resources for the services or equipment you need.
	Consider what services might be available through county and state programs. Text, call, or look for these services online. (Most states have a website listed with the number "211" and the name of the state. For example, mine would be "211 Wyoming.")
	Find out about Uber and Lyft services in your area. Lyft may provide free or discounted rides to doctor appointments if you contact them through your state's 211 number.
	Does your community have a hospice program? The wonderful staff and volunteers at most hospices are available to help in all sorts of ways, from monitoring or checking on a patient's health to picking up a gallon of milk. Find out what help they can provide and if your loved one qualifies for any of their services. Check online for the nearest hospice program at The National Hospice Locator website: www.nationalhospicelocator.com.
	Is there a precooked meal delivery service near you? Often called Meals on Wheels, or a similar name, the costs are low per meal and delivered to the door.
	Ask for helpful recommendations from your doctor and nurse.

	Talk to the social worker at the hospital, who will be aware of support services in your area.
	Remember that many grocery stores and supercenters offer online shopping with pickup and delivery services.
	Know that you can arrange pickup or delivery of restaurant meals through services such as Door Dash.
	If you live in the U.S. and get your mail at a neighborhood kiosk, the U.S. Post office may deliver directly to your home for a small fee.
	If you will be out of town for an extended time, ask the post office to hold your mail until you are able to return and pick it up.
	If investigating all of the above items feels overwhelming, delegate someone to do the research, organize the information, and get back to you. Be sure to give them a deadline so that you get help when you need it.

Look how many resources you've considered already for getting help. You're doing great!

WORKSHEET - CHILDREN

For children directly affected by a loved one's illness or injury, this time is especially sensitive. A survey of caregivers of patients and professionals made the following suggestions. Which ones will you try?

	Have dinner together.
	Set up a regular routine.
	Notify the school, church, and activity leaders about what's going on the child's life.
	Be as open and honest as possible about your loved one's needs and prognosis without scaring them.
	Use the name of the illness (cancer, a heart attack, etc.) and where on the body it is located.
	Reassure them that this illness isn't contagious. (Unless doctors have indicated otherwise.)
	Let them know how the illness may affect them or change their lives in specific ways.
	Give them a few chores to help with the sick person.
	Depending on their ages, consider taking them to certain doctor or treatment appointments.
	If it's allowed, bring them along on hospital visits.
	Suggest, if possible, frequent phone calls with the sick person.
	Remember that using Facetime can provide visual reassurance.
	Opt for texting, which may be easier for the patient than phone calls.
	Reassure children with extra hugs and kisses.
	Encourage them to share their feelings.
	Play games with them or watch funny or silly movies.
	Seek professional mental health support for them as needed.
	If your ill loved one happens to be a child, consider contacting Make A Wish for help.

List other ideas, below, as they arise to help you remember them:

WORKSHEET - PETS

When a loved one becomes ill or receives a sudden diagnosis, many of us will turn to our pets as members of the family. (In my case, I couldn't imagine getting through the ups and downs of Larry's illness without our beloved corgis.) Pets provide comfort and love when we most need it.

But it's important to remember that pets have their own needs, which can get disrupted with the sudden demands of caregiving. What arrangements are necessary for your pet's welfare?

	Day care. (When Larry had infusions, our corgi puppy, Smarty, went to doggy day care to run off his excess energy. Smarty would curl up and nap with Larry afterward.)
	Boarding your pets at a kennel or pet sitter's home.
	A house sitter or the services of a pet sitter who comes to your home.
	A neighbor or family member to feed, water, and let your dogs outside or clean a litter box or bird cage, etc.
	The veterinarian's phone number and clinic address for when you're gone:
	Instructions for any medication your pet requires:
	Feeding directions:
	The name of your pet's preferred food and treats:
	Any upcoming appointments, such as grooming:

SEVEN

Patient Comfort

When caring for an ailing loved one, think kindness, kindness, kindness! Patient comfort involves many considerations that include providing entertainment, depending on the ability and needs of the sick person. Remember to be tolerant of those little things that irritate you. Staying good-natured increases everyone's pleasure.

Spending time with your loved one is one of the most important considerations:

- Reassure the person that you are there to help in any way you can.

- Sit beside them or lie down beside them.

- Comfort them by offering a back rub with a pleasant-smelling lotion.

- Pop a soft blanket in the clothes dryer for five minutes for a cozy feeling.

- Keep extra pillows available.

- Store a few popsicles in the freezer to use for a dry mouth—or just because.

- If they like TV, keep the remote in a place where they have easy access.

- Offer straws to make drinking easier for them.

- Opt for easy clothes like sweats that are simpler to change into and remove.

- Encourage your loved one to wear a comfy robe and slippers to make it easier to get out of bed and sit with others.

- Ensure your loved one wears pajamas made of a soft fabric that won't rub against their skin.

- Keeping his or her room cheerful with clean bed linens provides a sense of security.

- Remember that routines make life easier.

- Provide your loved one with comfort food that's also nutritious.

WORKSHEET - ENTERTAINMENT

Even if your loved one suffers from mental deterioration, it's important to help them have the best quality of life possible. Positive forms of entertainment will occupy his or her mind away from difficult circumstances. Depending on the person's mental and physical condition, you may need to "think outside the box" to find engaging ideas.

- Read to them. Look for books that are humorous or have a light feeling.

- Try audio books—as long as they aren't too fast-paced for them to follow.

- Turn on a podcast, which can provide a wealth of information and entertainment.

- Offer your loved one activities that require using his or her hands. Some examples include: squishing clay, stringing beads, or stacking Lincoln logs or building blocks.

- Paint with watercolors.

- Go for a drive in the country.

- Listen to music together.

- Visit with friends.

- Venture out for lunch or dinner at a quiet restaurant.

- Sit together and color in coloring books.

- Watch light movies—nothing sad or dramatic or frightening.

- Sit and hold hands .

- Take a short walk together daily, if possible.

- Encourage movement of some type—dancing, light exercises, or stretching.

- Sit outside in the sun.

- Sit on a park bench and watch for birds; listen to the sounds around you.

- Go to a coffee shop. (Larry enjoyed having a cup of mocha with a double shot of chocolate, so that became our special treat.)

- Turn an ordinary outing into an enjoyable event. Going for a haircut gains extra sparkle if you stop for an ice cream cone on the way home.

- Play bingo, card games, or board games.

- Work together on a puzzle.

- Toss a ball back and forth.

- Talk about memories of the past.

- Engage in sexual intimacy, depending on the situation and the patient. You may need to check with the doctor first.

Watch for new and unusual activities to share. Above all, remember that the journey doesn't have to be all sad. Stay positive, do the things your loved one enjoys, laugh when you can, and have fun. In its own way, this is a special time.

In the space below, build an activity list as you think of new ideas:

_____

_____

_____

_____

_____

_____

_____

_____

_____

_____

_____

_____

WORKSHEET - FOR TERMINAL PATIENTS

If your loved one is facing a terminal diagnosis, it's important to start having discussions about the future—as uncomfortable as these talks may be. The sooner you give your loved one a chance to express his or her final wishes, the more you can focus on cherishing the time you have left. What's more, your loved one will find it easier to articulate these wishes when they are relatively healthy, and both of you can be reassured that these difficult decisions have been made in advance.

The worksheet, below, provides a list of key questions to ask your loved one. In most cases, simple, one-or-two-word answers should be enough.

Will there be a service (a celebration of life, funeral, etc.)?
If there is to be a service, does your loved one have in mind the reciting of Bible verses, the playing of favorite music, or the presence of particular speakers at the event?
Does he or she wish to be cremated or buried in a casket?
Has he or she chosen a particular burial site or location for distributing the ashes? If so, where?
Does he or she wish to be an organ donor?
Is there a current will or estate plan in place?

EIGHT

Visitors

Once word gets out about your loved one's condition, friends and family will probably want to drop by for a visit. Some of these visitors can bring good cheer and joy to you and your loved one. Others may be the gloom-and-doom-types. You are not obliged to open your door wide for everyone in your circle, especially when your loved one is ill.

Keep in mind that part of your role is to manage these visits in the best interests of you and your loved one. You don't need to put up with negative people or those who think they know how you feel, even though they've never been in your place.

Ask your loved one how often they want to be with others. Some don't want many others around while they're resting and recuperating, while others might like to be distracted with lots of visitors. Sometimes, your loved one will feel too ill for visitors and you'll need to be the gatekeeper. You can address others' needs and requests in a way that works for both of you.

Here are a few ideas to help you with visitors you deem unwelcome:

- Don't invite these people to help you.
- Don't agree with their unsolicited or unsuitable suggestions.
- Let them leave a message when they call rather than talking to them directly. Alter your outgoing message as needed.
- Ignore upsetting texts or simply block them.
- If grouchy old Uncle Albert shows up at your doorstep and you feel you must let him in, do so. After ten or fifteen minutes, get up from your chair, thank him for coming, and walk him to the door.
- Tell an unwelcome visitor—even a family member—who is cranky, pushy, or demanding that you're sorry, but they are upsetting you or your loved one. Politely ask them to leave.

- If people show up at an inconvenient time, suggest a better time.

- Don't back down, even if they insist. Your loved one may be sleeping or you may have other plans.

- It's okay to request that people call before they drop in, allowing you to suggest a good time for their arrival.

- You may want to set times when you don't wish to be disturbed with phone calls, texts, or visits. Set up a schedule and spread the word with family and friends.

Visiting an ill person—especially one with poor prospects of surviving—can be painful and difficult. Prospective visitors might worry about an upcoming visit. How is their sick friend going to look? What will they talk about? Feelings like these can be uncomfortable for everyone. This is your chance to step in and try to make the best out of these visits.

When your visitor arrives, be prepared to introduce appropriate topics of conversation that can make the visit go more smoothly. Avoid controversial discussions about politics or religion, unless you know these topics won't cause hard or difficult feelings. Here are some neutral starter topics to keep the conversation flowing and reduce those initially uncomfortable sensations for your visitor:

- Current events (particularly light or entertaining ones)
- Reminiscing about past
- Planning a meal or activity together
- Stories about pets or children
- Emotions if appropriate and desired by the patient
- Sports scores or updates on teams
- A funny, upbeat story
- What's been going on at work (again, with a focus on lighthearted topics)

If your loved one brings up heavier subjects and decides he or she wants to talk about end-of-life care or final wishes, the emotional ups and downs of their condition, the illness itself, or what he or she still wants to do in the ensuing months or years, don't shy away from these topics. Encourage visitors to simply listen. Often ill people—particularly if they're terminal—are really just wanting to be heard.

Try to remain calm and project a sense of ease and openness with your visitor as a way to allay their anxiety. Even if you never use any of the suggested conversation starters, you'll feel more confident knowing you have some options.

WORKSHEET - CONVERSATION STARTERS

If you want to be even more prepared for visitors, make a list of your own conversation starters:

_____

_____

_____

_____

_____

_____

_____

_____

_____

_____

_____

_____

_____

_____

_____

_____

_____

NINE

Your Self-Care

Being the primary caregiver for someone you love is mentally and physically draining in ways you have yet to discover. The grief can weigh you down, and although there may be a good ending to your story, it may not turn out quite the way you want it to.

Way too many caregivers neglect basic care for themselves. We tend to think everything should be about the sick person, but that's not true. You need medical attention and breaks. No guilt allowed here! If you don't keep up with your mental and physical health, burn-out can get in the way of being able to do your job.

When you are caring for someone else, it's so easy to set aside your own health needs and tell yourself you'll get to them later. The following worksheet will remind you of ways to stay healthy and keep you on track. You can use this worksheet for reference as you sort out which appointments you need and what date you've booked them. As you attend these appointments, mark down when you did so. You can also make note of which appointments still need to be made.

These steps will ensure you're showing up in the best possible way to care for your loved one.

WORKSHEET - CHECK SHEET FOR YOUR PHYSICAL SELF-CARE

Date	Appointment
	Primary doctor
	Specialist
	Dental appointment
	Teeth cleaning
	Eye exam
	Mammogram (women)
	Prostate exam (men)
	Colonoscopy
	Wellness exam
	Shingles vaccination (ask your doctor about this)
	Covid vaccination
	Flu shot (ask your doctor about this)
	Other vaccinations as recommended by your doctor

WORKSHEET - SIGNS OF DEPRESSION

If you notice any of these symptoms, be sure to discuss them with your doctor. You could be experiencing early depression, a common result of caregiver burnout.

- Feelings of being unappreciated or overworked

- Gaining or losing weight

- Being cross and irritable with others

- Insomnia (and related fatigue) or oversleeping

- A deep sense of sadness

- A loss of interest in things you used to enjoy

- Regular frustration or hopelessness over a loss of control

- A sense of isolation from your usual activities, friends, and family

- Constant worrying

- Not being interested in taking care of yourself

- Abuse of alcohol or drugs, even prescription medications

- Feeling burned out

There is something called anticipatory grief, the grief that comes with mulling over an event that hasn't happened yet, but that comes with a hidden toll. Many caregivers are vulnerable to depression even before they lose a loved one. Reach out for help if you are experiencing any of the above symptoms or think you need it. You may benefit from general counseling or grief counseling at this time.

Know that you are not alone in this struggle. You deserve to take good care of yourself and to know that you're going to be alright.

TEN

Simple Things Matter

There are times when you simply do what needs to be done. You are a caregiver. Your loved one's life is important. It's sometimes easy to neglect your own care or to tell yourself you'll eventually get around to tending to your own needs.

One day in the midst of my caregiving duties, the neuro-oncologist's nurse called and told me that Larry had developed drug-induced diabetes. She said she would set me up with the supplies and guidance to give him his daily shots. I dreaded the idea. I was certain I couldn't give him injections, but there was no other option.

As I drove from the Flying Saucer Campground to the doctor's office, I repeated to myself over and over, "I can do this. I can do this. I can do this."

When I arrived, Nurse Mary showed me the syringes I would use to inject Larry's insulin. *Scary!* For some reason, I noticed her manicured fingernails. She kept them short and rounded with a coat of pale nail polish.

Looking down at my own hands and ragged nails, I was embarrassed and tried to hide them from view. But I'm sure she must have noticed. Although I hadn't always kept my nails polished, ordinarily, they looked trimmed and clean. For weeks, I hadn't paid any attention to them. It was a simple oversight, but added to the fact that my hair needed a cut and my clothes looked sloppy—I clearly appeared like someone who was neglecting herself. In a way, I'd given up trying.

I had been directing all my attention toward Larry and his illness, and I'd forgotten to take care of me. It happens so often to caregivers. You may be so tired at the end of the day that you let yourself go. Depression might be the root cause of your neglect, but you'll feel better if your nails are in decent shape, your hair is clean, and your clothes aren't the same ones you wore when you scrubbed the toilet yesterday.

With a little effort toward your own care, you'll feel happier and others will respond to you better. You'll even figure out you can do things like those dreaded injections. You might not enjoy it, but you can do it.

WORKSHEET - SIMPLE THINGS MATTER

Now is the time to tend to your personal wellness—especially while you have the opportunity. Schedule these self-care dates into your life for the month. Write the date or location where each will take place and make a commitment to showing up for yourself.

Date	Appointment
	Haircut or styling
	Exercise
	Manicure
	Massage (try to book at least one a month if possible)
	Entertainment break (go shopping, out to movies, coffee dates, etc.—aim to do this weekly)
	Meal break (splurge on takeout, meal delivery, or dining out—again, aim to do this weekly if possible)
	Personal cleanliness (ongoing)

ELEVEN

Positive Attitude

Until my husband got ill, I had never given much thought to the power of mind over matter. But one day when Larry was in Swedish hospital, his neuro-oncologist stopped by to visit him. I met the doctor in the hallway with a specific question in mind.

"What part does a positive mindset play in an illness?" I asked.

The doctor and I settled into a couple of tan faux leather chairs placed along the wall. He glanced in the direction of the rehab wing where Larry had been for over a week. Then he turned back to focus his eyes on me.

"I can tell you that a positive attitude makes a difference . . . How much?" He shrugged his shoulders. "I can't say it will save a person's life, but I do know that a negative attitude will kill him."

One of the most important things you can do to help yourself and your loved is to set the tone and attitude for your caregiving and to do so as quickly as possible. It's not easy when you're feeling sad about your loved one's prognosis, but in the long run you'll both benefit from the decision to remain upbeat.

The thing about any serious illness with poor statistics of survival or recovery is that you begin grieving at the start. At first, shock doesn't let you comprehend what has happened. Denial sets in. *He was fine a minute ago, so how could this be true?* While trying to process this shock and denial, you're now being asked to put your own grieving aside while you display a brave face for your loved one. No wonder caregivers struggle to take care of themselves.

It might help to remind yourself that your feelings are natural, and may change while you're putting in all that effort to remain positive. Keep in mind the five stages of grief a person experiences, which will likely fluctuate within any given day or week:

- Denial

- Anger

- Bargaining

- Depression

- Acceptance

Of course grief doesn't occur in a straight line. You can't say to yourself, *I'm in denial now. It will be replaced by anger, then bargaining.* Grief skips around. Today you may feel denial and next week bargaining, only to return to denial the following week. It's also possible that you won't feel all the stages. Various people don't. At some point, acceptance finds its place.

But here's the thing: just as your loved one benefits from your upbeat attitude, caregivers who keep a positive outlook will also move more peacefully through the stages of grief. Keep in mind the following:

- Your loved one is much more likely to give up if you are negative.

- Giving up is contagious.

- You will better weather your loved one's illness by being positive.

The ill person may suffer a decline in mental functioning, and you may deeply grieve for the once strong, vital person who is now disappearing before your eyes. Watching your loved one struggle to live through rigorous treatments and unpleasant side effects, while contemplating your abrupt change in circumstances, is enough to bring anyone down. It is easier to succumb to sadness and worry, after all, than it is to fight those tendencies.

Remember, your loved is also going through the grieving process. You may not be in the same stages at the same time, but your loved one's grieving includes contemplating his or her own death or disability. The more you can remain positive now, the more you'll be able to reassure yourself later that you offered the best mental medicine for both of you throughout this difficult period.

WORKSHEET — WHAT WILL HELP YOU REMAIN POSITIVE?

It takes a deliberate effort to maintain a positive attitude while grieving and caregiving for a loved one. Here are a few ways to do so. Circle the activities you're most likely to practice.

- Avoid unhelpful, pessimistic people.

- Avoid negative news. You have enough to worry about without adding to it.

- Read and search for encouraging articles.

- Engage in reading light books and articles that make you smile. Joke books are great.

- Watch humorous movies or shows.

- Look for the good in situations whenever possible.

- Smile even when you don't feel like it. You will feel better.

- Try to stay away from Googling information on your loved one's disease. What you find may only make you feel worse—and there's a good chance the information isn't up to date or accurate. Wait to let your doctor help you better understand the illness.

- Do not say "what if . . ." and name something horrible that could happen to your loved one.

- Talk with a friend or family member who will help you maintain a positive attitude.

- Enjoy some dark chocolate.

- Go for a walk. Take a break every few yards. Breathe deeply in and out three times. Clear your mind of everything but what you can see, hear, feel, touch, and smell.

- Remind yourself that you can survive this time. It won't last forever.

- Sit on the floor with your cat or dog and stroke it for a few minutes.

- Think of what used to make you happy. Do you love the smell of fresh flowers on your table? Buy colorful ones. Grocery stores often sell cheerful but inexpensive flowers.

- If it's near a holiday, put out some simple decorations.

- Wear a pink shirt instead of that dull-colored one. A T-shirt with a clever saying? How about a happy one for your loved one?

- Make nachos or enjoy a snack of cookies and milk just because you feel like it. If your loved one can join you, rejoice.

- Live in the moment. Right now.

- Close your eyes, sit back, and listen to music that you love.

- Hold hands with your loved one. It is the best feeling for you both.

- Think of something different rather than focusing on the things distressing you. Make it a positive thought.

- If you're having dark thoughts, change your point of view.

- Exercise along with a TV or streaming show.

- Retain a sense of humor. Attempt to see the silly side of incidents.

- Dance to some fast music.

- Practice deep breathing: inhale slowly and let your breath out for an extra beat or two while you try to get your belly button to sink into your backbone.

- Take short breaks throughout the day.

- Drink a cup of tea and thumb through a magazine.

- Get a massage—even just a foot or shoulder massage if you're short on time.

- Grow or develop new interests—or begin to investigate these at least.

- Work on an art project.

How many of the above items did you circle? _____

List other things you've thought of that might help you stay positive:

_____

_____

_____

_____

_____

_____

_____

_____

_____

_____

_____

_____

All of the above items may help stop negative thoughts in their tracks! After all, your mind can only hold one thought at a time. When you replace negative thoughts with positive ones, you're developing a healthy habit to sustain you through difficult times.

One day, after Larry had been in Swedish Hospital's ICU for a few days, I sat beside him on a straight-backed chair. He lay in a drug-induced coma. His temperature was up, so the nurse had removed all his clothing and draped a single sheet over the lower part of his body for privacy. Both of his arms were bound to the bed rails. Negative thoughts filled my head. I didn't want others to see him in such a helpless condition. Would he even survive?

My eyes began to fill with tears, but before the tears rolled down my face, I got out of the chair and walked over to the door where I could see the nurses' station. I wondered how nurses could do such a vital job, day after day. Some of their patients didn't live. Thank goodness they arrived for each shift and used their skills to help others. When I thought about the nurses, my negative emotions turned to gratitude.

It's easy to feel down and discouraged in the moment. The future is uncertain. All the plans you had are falling apart. Life is not the same, and it may never be again.

It's alright to cry. Crying is a good release from built-up stress and frustration. It rids you of part of that tension. _You're going to be okay._

At the end of each day, write down one positive thing you noticed or that happened during the day. It can be anything you're grateful for, but try to find something different each day. Use ten or fewer words to describe it. Writing down these grateful thoughts before bed tends to relax you.

While caring for Larry, I was sometimes too exhausted to write, so instead, I replayed the positive experience in my mind. It's one of the techniques I still use when I can't go to sleep.

WORKSHEET - SOMETHING GOOD HAPPENED TODAY

Date	Occurrence

TWELVE

Hope

As long as you have hope to hang your emotions upon—even while your loved one is stuck in bed—the sky looks bluer, and it's easier to smile. Your facial muscles turn your lips up and reduce the frown lines on your forehead. Smiling helps you have hope for the future. Hope is related to a positive attitude.

We tend to consider hope in medical terms as a cure for an illness. Think about the advances in medical research each year. When Larry was sick, one of our hopes was that even though his current treatment might not be the answer, every day that he lived meant that the medical field was one day closer to finding a remedy for his cancer. Each stable blood test or good MRI or a day when he felt better was a reason for hope. We'd celebrate these days with ice cream.

There's that kind of external hope for the small wins, and then there is the hope that an ill person may have of being able to do something they loved doing once more.

For example, Larry loved living in the country and running his tractor all around the place. His John Deere was a source of pride. One of the main things he used it for was to keep our lane—from the house to the state road—in drivable condition. Although he wasn't allowed to operate a vehicle, I didn't think to say anything about his tractor. One day, I heard him start it. When I looked out the door, he was fulfilling one of his hopes—to level the road again. The look of concentration on his face and the resulting smile when he finished was proof that his hope of being able to operate his tractor again was fulfilled. I didn't think of standing in his way.

The reassurance you give your loved one that you will stay by them and that you still love them is critical to their emotional well-being. Let them know how important they have been to you. Talk about the things they have accomplished in their life. Isn't that giving them the hope of leaving a positive legacy?

When the future looks grim, it's a difficult balance between the hard facts of an illness and keeping hope alive. Yet look for the good in all that you can. Laugh together about anything and everything that hits the two of you as funny. Enjoy the time you have left. Each day that brings a feeling of happiness keeps hope alive for another day.

Hope isn't going to remove the pain you feel if the illness is terminal, but it will help you cope with it. Not only do you need reassurance, but the sick person needs hope to continue the journey.

WORKSHEET - HOPES AND DREAMS

What are your hopes and dreams? Go wild!

_____

_____

_____

_____

_____

_____

_____

_____

_____

_____

_____

_____

_____

_____

_____

_____

_____

_____

THIRTEEN

Faith

Along with hope, faith may offer solace during this troubling time—both for you and your ailing loved one. If you already have a connection with God, it may become stronger while you're caring for your loved one. For those who don't go to church each Sunday, perhaps your faith originates with the sense of wonder you feel when you view flowers, the sunrise, a child, or a newborn animal. Some people find a stronger connection to God (or a higher power) while in the mountains or on the water. Wherever you go to get the reassurance of that higher power, know there is love surrounding you.

Even in this age when many people question the idea of a God, it is not uncommon to reach out for spiritual reassurance as we edge closer to death ourselves. Likewise, those without a connection to a higher power might begin to think of it more at this time. While caring for a person you feel great tenderness towards, you may find comfort with a spiritual connection.

Through meditation, you may find reassurance and strength to continue to care for your loved one. Having faith while you struggle with the difficulty of tending to a cherished person can bring comfort. It brought me reassurance that I wasn't alone while Larry was sick.

When Larry died, I was humbled to realize that no matter what I did or wanted or how much money was available for a cure, a higher power was still in charge. To me, that was God.

No matter what your spiritual beliefs, you may suffer less from depression if you find a form of faith to lean upon. Your faith may weaken when there are downturns in the sick person's condition. If that happens, you can't change the disappointment, but don't let go of your faith. Continue to love and care. If you believe in a higher power, let it lead you forward.

WORKSHEET - YOUR HIGHER POWER

In a few words, write about your connection to a higher power.

_____

_____

_____

_____

_____

_____

_____

_____

_____

_____

_____

_____

_____

_____

_____

_____

_____

FOURTEEN

Resilient People

Resilient people don't think of themselves as victims. They know their journey through grief will end. These strong people act and think in different ways, which helps them get through the rough times.

See if you can adapt the following qualities to your situation:

Resilient people know that difficult things happen. Suffering is a part of life. They know they're not alone. Instead of asking "Why me?" they ask the question, "Why not me?" The illness is going to happen to a certain number of people, why not me? Why not my loved one?

Resilient people know where to focus their attention. They spend time on the things they can change, not on what they can't. They are flexible, and they understand that it's easier to be negative because we're wired to be that way. Staying positive takes constant work, and they're willing to put in that work.

Resilient people think about their actions. Will having another glass of wine help me or harm me? Thinking like this gives them some control over their lives and it helps them make healthier decisions in their own best interests.

Choose to live your life.

Don't focus on what you don't have. Focus on and be grateful for what you do have. Think of the good things in your life at the end of each day. Being able to find the good can be powerful—even life-changing.

WORKSHEET

Use this page to name one thing you're grateful for at the end of each day. You'll not only find this practice lifting your spirits, but you'll enjoy looking back at your reflections on the days when it's harder to remember what you're grateful for.

Date	Today I'm grateful for...

FIFTEEN

Acceptance

One of the saddest aspects of caregiving is watching your loved one slowly move away from you. There isn't a magic wand to make this process of loss any easier. It's a hurt, a canker that festers in your mind and body. Loneliness may fill much of your internal void.

My lifelong mate lost the ability to drive, read, write, watch movies, and so much more. There was no way for me to make it right or help him hang onto life. I had to realize how helpless I was—that even though I had bought into the idea I could will myself into having everything I wanted, my desires had limits. In the big picture, we aren't the final decision makers.

The day may arrive when death is near and your loved one is leaving you. How do you prepare for a life without him or her? Is there any way to really be ready? Yes, you may have been the caregiver for a number of months or years, and you may have been grieving for all that time, but have you accepted what's to come in the end? Is that even possible?

Acceptance of my reality did not come to me until the morning Larry died in hospice. I could not imagine being separate from him. I knew in my mind that things had to change as he got weaker each day, but my heart had not accepted it. Had I gone back to the grief stage of denial?

Even though you may feel the truth, it doesn't mean you won't stop questioning the cause of the illness or accident or mulling over what could or should have been. Was it caused by genetics or something else? Often, there is no definitive answer. You have to let it go and go on with your life. You are strong. You can do this. I did. And I'm infinitely grateful to know this is possible.

SIXTEEN

Denial and Bargaining

Denial and bargaining are two stages of grief we've already identified. Not everyone goes through all five stages, but for those who do (as mentioned earlier), they tend to skip around from one stage to the next. If your loved one's condition is terminal or even potentially terminal, grieving may begin while the person is still alive.

To me, denial and positive thinking went together like a pair of jeans and a shirt. They formed a protective shield around me. Since I couldn't control what was happening, denial blocked my gaze on a negative future. Positive thoughts and hope worked to keep me from falling into a black pit of anxiety. By including art activities and journaling, my stress level allowed me to function in an acceptable manner. I rarely thought of Larry leaving me. His death was something I couldn't comprehend. In this instance, I found myself grateful for this particular stage of grief.

Denial is the mind's natural defense system, a way of coping with a seemingly unbearable possibility. Since your loved one is still living, you may not even recognize being in denial.

Bargaining is another natural thought process for making yourself feel better. It allows you to cope with the pain and sense of helplessness. It can involve making deals with yourself to do something better or differently in exchange for a better outcome. While bargaining can also be an extension of denial, if the promises are practical and you commit to keeping them, then this type of deal making can actually be helpful.

For instance, you might say to yourself, "if my loved one has good blood test results tomorrow, I'll bake him a cherry pie." If the results are positive, you would need to get into the kitchen and start that cherry pie—an activity that might make you feel better and will certainly cheer up your loved one. This is an example of working with the stages of grief in a positive way.

Negotiating through grief can also work against our mental well-being. You might attempt to strike a deal with a higher power in the hopes of getting a positive result, asking God to spare your loved one, for instance, if you agree to attend church every Sunday. Of course, life doesn't work that way, and leaning too heavily into this form of prayer can be dispiriting and even heartbreaking. In the end, we aren't in control of the final outcome.

Instead, you can shift your focus from something you can't control to something you can. What's something you and your loved one would enjoy doing together while you can?

Think of the goodness around you. Remind yourself that you are going to be alright.

SEVENTEEN

Guilt Feelings

The monumental responsibility given to caregivers can cause feelings of guilt that destroy their sense of peace (and negatively affect their loved ones). Caregiver guilt often comes from feeling that you should do everything yourself and that what you're doing just isn't enough. You could be anxious, for instance, that you've made a mistake in administering medication at the wrong time or forgetting it entirely. A list for crossing off pill times will remedy that problem. But before you make that list, tell yourself your loved one is lucky to have you—and that you are giving him or her the best you possibly can. Know that when the load becomes too much to bear, it's okay to call for professional help.

This might be a good time to do a self-assessment. Does doing your best still not sound good enough? Are you struggling with the fear your idle mistakes could lead to something dire? It's important to step back and assess how much guilt you're carrying while caring for your loved one. Imagine that his or her health has slipped and he or she is confined to the hospital for a few days.

How might you feel?

- Would you blame yourself for this sudden downturn?

- Fret or lose sleep because your caregiving has been shown to be deficient?

- Or would you understand that this is a chance to give the load to those more competent and qualified?

Freeing yourself from accountability for a few days can be like eating a giant piece of chocolate cake. The ultimate indulgence. Someone other than you has arrived to take charge of everything about the patient. The experts will know what to do; your loved one's needs are in good hands. Finally, you can relax.

Reaching out for help and finding a way to cut ourselves some slack sounds easy, but sometimes we let our guilt take over our common sense. Does that sound like you? To find out, circle the best answer, below.

You don't have the kind of coffee your loved one wants. Do you:

- Serve what you have and promise to buy the favored brand for tomorrow?

- Feel guilty and blame yourself for not buying his favorite brand?

- Run right out and buy some of the right brand?

- Gruffly give her a cup of whatever you have or give her nothing?

If you've said yes to any of the above, it's time to stop and take a breath. Since you can't do all and be all, remind yourself that you're doing all you can. Don't beat yourself up for neglecting the small stuff. Buy the special coffee the next time you shop.

Measure your guilt meter in another circumstance. Imagine that a friend asks you to go to a movie. You haven't been anywhere for relaxation for three weeks. You really want to go, maybe you even want to grab a quick snack after the movie. You make arrangements for someone to sit with your loved one, but you're pondering the fact that he or she hates it when you leave.

Circle yes or no to the following questions:

- Should you go? Yes No

- Would you go? Yes No

- Would you feel guilty? Yes No

In considering your answers, keep in mind that part of your responsibility as a caregiver is to take care of yourself. Your job is to make your loved one's life the best it can be under the circumstances. How he or she improves medically ultimately isn't up to you.

Here are some positive suggestions, below, to lessen any feelings of guilt:

- Remember, you are doing the best you can, especially if you weren't trained for this situation.

- No one person can do everything. Besides caregiving, you may have children, a job outside the home, laundry, your pets, the house. The list goes on. It's okay to hire or ask for some help.

- Self-care is not selfish. If you don't take care of yourself, you won't be able to care for anyone else. An occasional break, like a movie with a friend, is important to stop the stress from making you ill.

- You aren't responsible for improving the prognosis of your loved one. You can't fix this! However, following the doctor's directions is your responsibility; this is usually in the realm of a caregiver's capabilities. But when it isn't, reach out for help.

- When pondering the random cruelty of your loved one's situation, avoid thinking, "why not me?" So much of life is unexpected and impossible to explain. You aren't the sick one, but you have the opportunity to help someone you love feel a little better. That's the silver lining amid the misfortune.

- If things go well for a day or you see even modest improvement in your loved one's demeanor, celebrate those moments with an ice cream cone, a special coffee, or some other small treat.

- Realize you are doing important work. Every small gesture matters. Think of it this way: will you ever do anything more important than helping someone go through the last days, months, or years of life?

- Be grateful for all the good things you enjoy. Maybe it's as simple as getting through the day without losing your temper or crying every hour. Those little victories add up to a larger one. Caregiving for someone you love isn't for the faint of heart.

To be honest, even though I did as much as I could for my husband, I occasionally experience pinpricks of guilt. I tell myself, "I could have done this better" or, "why didn't I do that for him?" In these moments, I stop and shake my head. There's no point in dwelling on it now. It's all in the past, and the reality is, I did my best. Keep your positive frame of mind alive. It helps everyone around you—and you'll need to return to it again and again as you process your grief.

EIGHTEEN

More Feelings

One of the best ways to avoid the inevitable sense of isolation that comes with caregiving is to reach out to others about your situation. But it's easy to neglect this step when you're busy tending to your loved one. Does this sound like you? Have you been able to talk about the future and your feelings with your loved one and at least one other individual?

If not, remember to reach out to an understanding friend or even a therapist. A minister can also be a good person to meet with to help calm your fears.

Each illness is unique to the person facing it, and every caregiving situation can vary from others. Facing the unknown takes tremendous courage. The initial fear of a diagnosis, and acknowledging what's required of you, can bring sudden, unwelcome changes. It's critical to be able to talk openly with others as you adjust to this unexpected upheaval.

Being patient and maintaining a sense of humor will also go a long way toward making this new situation bearable. A caregiver-friend once said, "Thank goodness I've kept my sense of humor—or I'd kill him." I knew she didn't mean it, but we both had a good laugh over that.

As you process these new, difficult feelings aloud, consider additional ways to deal with the loss of things you can no longer control. As you do, remember that these feelings are ultimately short-lived. You will get through this time. You won't always feel like this.

- Cry when you need to.

- Focus on short-term plans.

- Journal about your feelings.

- Talk to your support system or team.

- Stay active.

- Listen to soothing music.

- Take a walk in a garden.

- Treat yourself in some minor way.

Don't be so hard on yourself. You're doing the best you can. That means you're doing great!

WORKSHEET - FEELINGS

The role of caregiver can bring up a raft of emotions, all of them important to note and process as they arise. The following worksheet cites a series of emotions you may feel from the first signs of your loved one's illness and continue through his or her treatment. You'll be better equipped to manage this time by writing down a few words about each feeling as you encounter it. As you do, review earlier sections of this workbook for positive ways to tackle these feelings. Understanding and addressing what your mind is telling you helps free your thoughts, rather than letting them bottle up and veer toward worry or a sense of hopelessness.

Loneliness

As a caregiver, you are performing an act of love for your cherished one. But that love can feel one-sided at times and give way to a unique kind of loneliness, particularly as you spend a few solitary minutes trying to gather your thoughts. You may think no one else understands what you're going through—and in some ways, you may be right.

How do you deal with loneliness?

Fear

No matter how hard you try to avoid it, you will face moments of fear—fear of the unknown, fear of your own imaginings. Try to set fear aside and live for right now.

What are some ways you can combat fear when it strikes you?

Happiness

Not all of this journey is filled with misery and sadness. Depending on your loved one's condition, there may be lots of things you can still do together. Whenever possible, I took Larry somewhere—even if it was just a drive around town. One day he said, "I'm not unhappy." And, at that moment, I realized I wasn't either.

If there's a good day, and you feel happy, what was the reason for that? How can you give the two of you more happy days?

Anger

Anger stems from many places, including from impatience. After you've been asked what time it is for the twentieth time in an hour, it's hard to be patient. But it's so important to be patient nonetheless. Remember that medication can make your loved one say things he or she wouldn't ordinarily say. Your patient didn't want this illness or accident and neither did you.

Describe your anger.

Regret

We all have regrets about things we have done or said or didn't do or say. Those actions are in the past, and they can't be redone. It takes negative energy to look backwards at your doubts.

Write your major regrets below, then cross them out as if you've thrown them away. Be rid of them.

A sense of peace

You might have feelings of peace, especially if you live mentally in "day-tight containers," without the past or worry of tomorrow to bother you. These moods could be fleeting, but by being able to be with the sick person, you can appreciate a moment of quiet intimacy. Sitting without needing to speak brings such a sense of closeness.

What causes those moments of peace for you? How do they feel?

| |
| |
| |
| |
| |
| |

Disappointment

You're not alone. Disappointment hits everyone. Maybe not today, but sometime. From pondering the trips you can't take to missed dinners with friends, you're going to need to deal with your feelings of loss.

Look back at the suggestions found in this workbook to help you accept the hard choices you must make. Write about some of your disappointments and say why they upset you. What can you do to reduce the unhappiness you feel?

| |
| |
| |
| |
| |
| |
| |

Abandonment

While your attention is directed toward someone special who needs your care, your friends will move on with their own lives. It isn't that they don't care, but they will continue going to movies, taking trips, and dining out. They may make new friends to do these activities with since you are no longer available. It's disappointing, but it's the reality of life. You'll still be friends, but that friendship will change.

How can you make yourself feel better about these unexpected changes?

Self-Pity

Instead of feeling sorry for yourself as a newfound caregiver, take a minute to acknowledge that you are hurting. Life doesn't seem fair. You're lost and afraid. Remember that in this moment, lots of others in the world are suffering too. It's natural to feel self-pity during challenging times. Take a few minutes to feel sorry for yourself.

How are you going to get through this situation without making yourself a victim?

Sadness

Because of the seriousness of your loved one's condition, you're bound to feel an underlying sadness. The sorrow is there, and it colors everything else in your life if you let it. That sadness may be the grief of watching your loved one struggle to survive, and realizing you can't slow down or change the outcome.

What can you can do to deal with melancholy? (If the sadness seems overwhelming or unmanageable, seek medical help right away.)

NINETEEN

Relapse

If there is anything that breaks your heart nearly as much as the original diagnosis, it must be a relapse. Everything is going well. You tell yourself that there's no reason for circumstances to change. You have done your best for your loved one, and that's when you begin to ease up. Then it happens: you go to the doctor and the test results reveal the awful truth—your reprieve is over.

After an intense fight for survival, it's back again, and you feel ill-equipped to keep your spirits up on behalf of your loved one. How can you reassure him or her when the news is so crushing? What's going to happen next?

- Find out from the doctor what choices are available.

  o The situation has changed, so the treatment options may also have changed. New medications may be available. Surgery previously considered impossible may now be a reasonable option.

- Go to a quiet place with your loved one to discuss what he or she wants.

  o Your loved one may be too tired to want to continue with the fight. It might not be your choice, but this isn't your body or your life.

  o Your loved one's age will affect the decision the two of you make.

  o If your loved one isn't mentally able to tell you his or her choice, what do you think he or she would want? (In this case, is his or her medical directive available?)

- Consider: what do you want?

- What is your loved one's expected quality of life?

- After you have made a decision together, meet with the doctor and relay that decision.

- Begin treatment again, or if your loved one doesn't want any more treatment, respect his or her wishes. This isn't about you as much as it is about them and their conscious choice.

You have done the best that you can for your loved one. Now you must be courageous enough to continue the course. If treatment starts once more, remain positive. If your loved one chooses to end treatment, respect that. Share your love and kindness.

You may not be a hundred percent certain that you or your loved one have made the right decision. Do the best that you can with the information available to you.

Don't second-guess yourself. Move on. You're doing great!

TWENTY

Respite Care

Primary caregiving is exhausting—emotionally and physically. Being able to get away for a few hours every day or two is part of keeping your sanity. If your loved one needs constant care and a friend or family member can't spell you off, reach out to a service that can provide someone to sit with your loved one while you take a break.

If you do find yourself in the position of needing to hire someone from a reputable service, ask about the person they plan to send. Depending on your loved one's comfort level and previous experiences, the age and sex of the caregiver can be important. Will that type of person work for your loved one?

There may come a time when you are drained to the point of needing more than a few hours to rejuvenate. Respite care gives you a break for several days to recover the energy you might have lost.

Your budget may be a factor. If you are in the U.S., you may need to pay out of pocket for this service, depending on your private insurance coverage or the requirements of Medicare or Medicaid.

The usual options for respite care include the following (listed by cost):

- A relative or friend who stays twenty-four hours a day

- An adult day-care facility with someone else doing the night shift

- A trained professional who comes into the home and stays twenty-four hours a day

- A nursing home, assisted living, or memory care unit

- A service provided through hospice homes

I attended a lecture on respite care where attendees were told to take their patient to one of the homes even if he or she didn't want to go. After I left the lecture, I decided to talk to Larry about the idea. My first suggestion of having his brother or cousin come stay with him for a few days wasn't agreeable to him.

Next, I mentioned the idea of him going to a nursing home while I made a trip to Casper because he was so fragile. We hadn't been home for several months. Tears rolled down his cheeks into his beard, and he said, "Please don't leave me."

I thought of all the time he'd spent in the hospital, and I didn't have the heart to leave him for even a few days. Since I didn't really want to be away from him either, we dropped the subject.

In our case, respite didn't provide an immediate solution. It isn't for everyone. But it's certainly worth considering. A respite break can make all the difference in your ability to continue to care for your loved one at home. And when you return, your stress level will be lower, making everything more manageable again for both of you.

If you decide to take the ill person to a hospice or skilled nursing home for a few days of rest for yourself, how will you do it? Circle the most likely way you'll handle it:

- Announce that your loved one is going and pack his or her bag.

- Discuss the idea calmly with your loved one, explaining why you need the rest.

- Offer some alternatives to a nursing home or other hospital-like setting.

- Reconsider your suggestion if your loved one grows upset.

- Think about your loved one's recent hospital stays, and if they didn't go well, choose not to mention the idea of respite care at all.

WORKSHEET - FREE DAY ACTIVITIES

If you've sought or found respite for your loved one, you now have a few free days for yourself. List five things you'd like to do during those days. Then, number them from one to five in order of importance and aim to do as many as you can.

Order	Things I'd like to do:

TWENTY-ONE

What is an SNF?

Larry's doctor admitted him to Swedish hospital on a Friday. On Saturday, Dr. A. came to see us. "Larry will need to be admitted to an SNF in a day or two," Dr. A. said. "He's too sick to go home with you. Insurance won't let him stay in the hospital longer than that."

After Dr. A. left, I asked a nurse what the doctor meant by "SNF."

"There are three kinds of skilled nursing facilities—SNFs," she explained. "They're called that because the patient needs more specialized care than what's offered in a normal nursing home or assisted living environment. They offer physical, occupational, and speech therapy, as well as other things."

I nodded to let her know I was listening.

"There are three varieties of SNFs around here. They're all at nursing homes. At one type, if the patient doesn't want to go to therapy, they don't push them. The second kind encourages the patient to get the therapy without insisting. But the third kind doesn't take no for an answer. They expect the person to participate in the therapy with the goal of going home."

There wasn't any doubt in my mind. Larry would go to the third type of SNF. I made the decision because he wasn't conscious enough to help me decide. He attended the SNF in question and did his therapy. Then, even though his doctor hadn't expected him to survive, at the end of seven weeks, Larry walked out of the SNF. After that, I developed a new appreciation for SNFs.

If you want your loved one to go to an SNF for a short-term stay, he or she must have a doctor's recommendation. SNFs are often located in dedicated wings or floors of nursing homes.

Insurance may pay for this type of care for a certain number of days, depending on how well the patient improves with care. If the patient progresses, the insurance coverage may be extended past the initial approval time.

Medicare covers the cost of SNFs for a defined amount of time. Among qualifying admissions is the provision that a person has stayed in a hospital during the previous thirty days.

The home's billing department or admissions person can help you work through any payment issues.

Although attending an SNF can mark an endpoint for some people, your loved one can progress toward being able to go home. If your loved one goes to such a place, make sure you are there frequently for support and encouragement, just as you were when your loved one was in the hospital.

Look for the good in this experience. It remains a happy memory for me.

TWENTY-TWO

Sleep: It's Critical

Caregiving is a demanding job, and if your situation is long-term, getting enough sleep is vital.

Sleep experts recommend getting seven-to-nine hours of rest daily to help keep your strength up. Naps and the hours you sleep in bed are all considered part of your daily count. While short naps work well, long ones make it more difficult to fall asleep at night.

If you're in a long-term caregiving situation, take the two-week survey, below, to see if you're getting adequate rest. Did you count that fifteen-minute nap you took when you sat down to read but dozed off?

WORKSHEET - SLEEP TRACKING

Day of Week	Hours of Sleep	Days of Week	Hours of Sleep
Sunday		Sunday	
Monday		Monday	
Tuesday		Tuesday	
Wednesday		Wednesday	
Thursday		Thursday	
Friday		Friday	
Saturday		Saturday	
Week one total		Week two total	

How'd you do?

WORKSHEET - IMPROVING SLEEP

Here are some ideas you can try to improve your sleep. Put a check beside each one that you've tried. Circle those you find most helpful.

	Develop a sleep schedule where you go to bed at the same time each night and get up at the same time each day.
	Try to get some exercise during the day, but not immediately before bed.
	Make your sleeping area conducive to sleep—cool, dark, quiet.
	Don' t eat heavy meals before bedtime.
	If you need a snack before bed, try peanut butter on whole grain toast or crackers or a piece of lean cheese on whole grain crackers.
	Avoid naps, especially long ones.
	Reduce caffeine and alcohol for several hours before bedtime.
	An hour before bedtime, turn off your cell phone. Read or journal instead.
	Try visualizing you're in a peaceful place or meditating by relaxing each body part.
	I frequently begin a story in my head. Usually after a few minutes, I fall asleep. The next night I start at the beginning once more with the same result. The story never gets finished. One day when I mentioned this routine to my mom, she told me she did the same thing and we both found this method helpful for getting to sleep.
	Before you go to bed, jot down what you need to do the next day so that you don't worry about forgetting it.
	Consult your doctor if sleeplessness is a severe problem.
	Consider respite care for your loved one. (See Chapter 20 on respite care.)

TWENTY-THREE

Practical Food Tips

Before I talk about healthy eating habits, I want to first stress the importance of staying hydrated. People who are sick often won't drink enough water. That's also true of caregivers. Dehydration can cause mental confusion, loss of strength, and headaches, as well as a whole host of other issues. Sweetened soda is not a substitute for water. Green tea is good, but water is best for both you and your loved one.

Here are a few healthy food tips for busy caregivers:

- **Watch sodium in pre-packaged meals.** The FDA recommends no more than 600 mg of sodium per serving in frozen meals and canned soups for them to be considered healthy. Meals with more sodium are still edible but may not be best for regular consumption, especially if you're managing blood pressure or heart health.

- **Use a slow cooker for low-effort meals.** Crockpots are a great option on hectic days filled with appointments. Try prepping ingredients the night before so you can simply turn on the crockpot in the morning and have dinner ready when you return.

- **Make a big batch of homemade soup.** Soup is comforting, versatile, and a great way to include vegetables and lean protein. Freeze leftovers in individual portions for easy meals later.

- **Keep a rotisserie chicken on hand.** It's a quick and affordable protein source that can be used in salads, sandwiches, wraps, or added to soups and pastas.

- **Check your supermarket deli.** Many delis offer ready-to-eat options like grilled vegetables, lean proteins, and salads. Look for dishes made with minimal sauces or added salt.

- **Don't overlook hospital cafeterias.** If you're spending long days at the hospital, the cafeteria may have healthier choices than fast food eateries or vending machines. Look for fresh salads, grilled items, or soups.

Even if you don't feel hungry, try to eat to keep your strength up. It's easy to get in the habit of eating fast food (I know, I love French fries) or candy bars for your meals. Try not to let yourself succumb, simply because it's quick and easy in the moment.

Cookbooks with easy, tasty recipes

These are certainly not the only cookbooks with fast, tasty recipes, but these are the ones I use and enjoy.

- *Fix-It and Enjoy-It 5-Ingredient Recipes* by Phyllis Pellman Good
- *Super-Fast Slow Cooking Cookbook* by Gooseberry Patch. (Each recipe uses only five ingredients)
- *Cooking Healthy* by Dr. Sally N. Hunt, PhD
- *Ultimate 4 Ingredient Diabetic Cookbook* by Dr. Sally N. Hunt, PhD. (Many recipes use fat-reduced or lower calorie ingredients, but if you don't have them, use what you do have. Although it's a diabetic cookbook, the recipes are great)

Websites with easy recipes

There are numerous websites with easy recipes for you to try. Here are a few I've used:

- Taste of Home (http://tasteofhome.com) This website has many options online and in print.
- Easy and Delish (https://www.easyanddelish.com) 130 easy five-ingredient-or-less recipes.
- Return to the Kitchen (http://returntothekitchen.com) 24 easy, four-ingredient-or-less, slow-cooker recipes.

Snacks

Snacking-on-the go takes on new significance for any busy caregiver. There isn't always time to have a nutritious meal, but it's always possible to find or make snacks with nutritional value. Aim for high-protein, low-fat, reduced sugar snacks with minimal processing, such as sliced apples dipped in peanut butter or cut-up vegetables with homemade hummus. Try to avoid chips and candy, although occasional dark chocolate with a minimum of seventy-percent cocoa is reported to be a good snack—and it's helpful for mental health!

Taking the time to give your loved one nutritious snacks offers an added bonus: if your children have just gotten home from school—or guests arrive unannounced—you have something on hand that everyone can enjoy together.

Good snack options

String cheese

Apples with peanut butter

Mixed nuts

Low sodium popcorn

Carrot strips

Hard-boiled eggs

Jerky (look for one with less sodium)

Cherry tomatoes with mozzarella

Energy bars (check the sugar level)

Oatmeal with fruit

Cheese with whole wheat crackers or fruit

Popsicles made with 100% fruit juice

Walnuts

Celery with cream cheese

Cottage cheese with fruit

Plain Greek yogurt with added fruit and nuts

Avocado on wheat toast

Last night's leftovers

Trail mix with dried fruit, nuts, and chocolate (in moderation, given the high calorie count)

TWENTY-FOUR

Talking It Out

If you are caring for a loved one with a serious or terminal illness, friends and family won't understand what you're facing unless they've been through a similar situation. They may be upset, even sympathetic. Without direct experience as a full-time caregiver for a family member—particularly a mate—they won't know what it's like to walk in your shoes.

For that reason, your doctor may encourage you to connect with caregivers of loved ones sharing the same or similar illnesses. There's a lot of empathy among a group with the common goal of helping each other get through a trauma in one piece. Without a magic wand to make the situation any easier, it helps to know you aren't alone.

What about chat groups? One day, a woman from the local cancer society called to suggest I join an online chat group with those whose loved ones suffered from glioblastoma brain tumors. The first time I joined in, the comments were all negative. During the two subsequent gatherings, the members primarily talked about friends who deserted them and the things they were missing out on because of the illness.

Those weren't the things I wanted to know. I'd hoped to learn about possible new activities to keep Larry entertained and interesting foods or recipes he might enjoy. Instead, this group was focused on venting—they had a different mindset than I did. These support group chats failed to uplift my spirits or provide positive feedback in a way I found helpful or hopeful. After a few days, I stopped visiting the chat room.

My experiences online were a lesson in finding the right fit for my circumstances. And just because my online support group experience didn't work for me, the concept of reaching out to others with the same struggles and concerns was something I still consider helpful. Many other caregivers have expressed their appreciation for the vital role support groups can play in breaking patterns of isolation and in building a sense of support in community.

Almost any kind of chat group can be located on the internet, particularly via Google or Facebook. You don't have to be dealing with the same illness, but do look for some similarities to your situation. One source of chat groups for caregivers can be found at www.caringbridge.org. You may also join a group specifically set up for the type of illness your loved one is faced with. If an online search doesn't yield what you are looking for, contact an office like the National Cancer Society that deals with the specific illness in question.

If you do find a suitable group, be sure to go to several sessions before deciding whether or not that group is a good fit for you. You may be lucky enough to find a chat group that offers exactly what you want and need: a group where you can share your insights while you learn from others. If you do, give yourself the relief of participating in it. There can be great comfort in connecting with others who know what you're battling.

WORKSHEET – WHAT TO LOOK FOR IN A CHAT GROUP

Before you jump into a chat group for caregivers, it's a good idea to have some idea of what you want to get out the group and what you might be able to contribute.

Here is a list of things to consider:

- Is the illness the same for each caregiver in the group? Does it matter if it isn't?

- Are your loved one's limitations similar enough to the sickness the group affiliates with to make you a good fit for the group?

- Does the group seem upbeat and positive most of the time?

- Do the members want to share helpful ideas and suggestions in answer to your questions?

- Do the chat times work with your schedule?

- What can you contribute to the group?

    1.

    2.

    3.

- What do you hope to gain from the group? List your top three wishes:

    1.

    2.

    3.

- How do you feel after attending one or two sessions? (Use your answer to gauge whether or not you'll continue to attend)

TWENTY-FIVE

Financial Help

When people receive traumatic health news, they typically aren't financially prepared, and their sudden inability to work and earn an income can become a problem. Thankfully, a range of resources are available for people to draw upon in the case of sudden injury or illness.

WORKSHEET - FINANCIAL HELP

	Apply for long-term disability. Ask your doctor for help. How soon your benefits will be awarded depends on how quickly the doctor does the paperwork and the severity of the illness. Although you won't receive the equivalent of a full salary, the extra income can be a huge help.
	If your loved one has suffered a work-related accident, apply for workers' compensation or employer insurance coverage as soon as possible. Ask the employer for help.
	Use your own savings in combination with other options.
	Check to make sure the doctor and facility you use are covered by your insurance company. If not, find out why. You may need to use a different doctor and hospital to meet policy requirements. Skilled nursing facilities (SNF) are usually covered by insurance, but you need to know in advance before relocating your loved one.
	Find out if the patient's insurance policy will pay for respite care while you take a short break. You may need to pay for this care yourself.

	Apply for food stamps and/or visit food pantries.
	Check your area for local services offering free or low cost food delivery services. Is there a program for seniors or ill persons in particular? Such a program may be called Rolling Meals, Meals on Wheels, or something similar.
	In the U.S., check with your county or state health department for caregiving assistance services in your area that offer help with house cleaning or running errands.
	Depending on your loved one's affliction, he or she may qualify for help from a range of non-profit organizations. For example, The National Brain Injury Alliance offers a variety of resources and services.
	Depending upon your income level, pharmaceutical companies may lower or subsidize the cost of necessary drugs. In some cases, they will donate them at no cost.
	When it comes to paying for accommodations, bigger hospitals often have a special price worked out with nearby hotels to reduce overnight stays for caregivers and/or patients. Sometimes, the hospital has access to low rental apartments. If a child is the patient, look for a local Ronald McDonald house.
	Ask your loved one's employer if employees have a vacation plan or sick day share system where each worker donates a day or two in advance as insurance against serious illness or injury. After the patient uses up his or her own sick days and vacation time, he or she may be able to draw from the shared bank of sick days.
	Set up a Go Fund Me account online or ask a friend to do it.
	Consider asking one or two ambitious friends to organize a benefit auction. Raffles, a sporting activity, a night of bingo, or anything which will bring people together to help can be a welcome source of ready cash.
	Churches are another source of temporary help, especially in providing meals, transportation, and other special needs.
	Does the patient qualify for a medical trial operated by a drug company? Ask your doctor. Call the drug company directly and ask about any programs they offer.
	Check with your local hospice about the possible provision of home care.
	In the U.S., talk with the billing department of your medical service provider. They may be able to work out a payment plan.
	While a loan may be a necessary last option, try to avoid mortgaging your house or vehicle in case repayment becomes difficult.

WORKSHEET - FINANCIAL MATTER WORKSHEET

If you are the caregiver for an ailing spouse, it's critical that you assume responsibility for household finances. Here are the financial matters you will need to know about (and have ready access to):

Where your money is kept	
Which banks hold your savings and/or investments	
Your brokerage accounts	
A calculation of your monthly budget based on your current assets and cash flow	
Life insurance policies (if any)	
Whether or not you have a mortgage on your home	
Information about your home insurance	
The current method of payment for taxes and/or your home mortgage	
Any outstanding loans, including vehicle loans	
The insurance agent for your vehicle coverage	

The current method of payment for your utilities and other monthly obligations	
Other financial obligations	
The location of your will and/or trust (if you have one)	
The location, key, and access information for your safety deposit box (if you have one)	
Contact information for your lawyer (if you have one)	
Information about your accountant and/or who has prepared state and federal taxes for you in the past	
Contact information for your financial planner (if you have one)	
Passwords	

TWENTY-SIX

Insurance Issues

If you're a caregiver relying on private insurance to fund your loved one's medical expenses, then chances are you're familiar with the struggle to get coverage for your claims. Of course, insurance companies are businesses. Their purpose, in addition to helping you, is to make a profit for their stockholders. They can't do that if they pay out more money than they take in, which might prompt them to take a strong stand on claim reimbursements.

Policies you purchase usually carry a disclaimer that cites the company's unwillingness to pay for experimental treatments. Your mental picture of the origin of these treatments may be of scientists working in a laboratory toward a cure. For the insurance company, experimental treatments are viewed as anything lacking FDA approval.

If your issue with the insurance company involves a procedure, your doctor or the hospital involved may have an insurance specialist whose job is to fight for a claim on your behalf. These people know how to work with the insurance company involved. Let them do their job.

However, with all the new advances in medicine, it may be difficult for your insurance company to keep up—and that's where you come in. You might be the first one to fight for coverage for a particular new medication for your loved one. The person who handles insurance for your doctor's office may be able to help you by contacting the insurance company and working with them on any new requests. The drug company may help with this also.

In some instances, none of these options work, and you may find yourself on your own in this fight. On average, the vast majority of denials of medical insurance coverage are not contested by claimants. For those claimants, fatigue—and the certainty they can't win—prevent them from going up against the business.

If you are part of that worn-out majority, refer back to Chapter 25 on Financial Help, and use as many of these options as possible that apply to your loved one. Be prepared for a hefty bill. In the effort to cover high medical costs, some people use up their savings and take out loans. They always run the risk these actions could result in bankruptcy.

Those who do fight insurance companies, have one thing in common. They become like a bulldog who has a sock in his mouth. He takes a firm bite and shakes his head back and forth without ever letting go.

Our insurance company denied coverage for the expensive drug effectively killing Larry's brain tumor. The drug in question did not have FDA approval for use with brain tumors, although it did have approval for use with other cancers. The pharmaceutical company had applied for FDA approval, but it would be nearly a year before the FDA granted it or rejected it.

In the interim, I decided to fight for Larry's right to receive the drug for two reasons: He was young—only sixty-two—and the drug had already shown remarkable power in killing the tumor. Filled with hope for my husband, I became a bulldog.

But even a stubborn bulldog must pick her battles. If you decide to fight an insurance denial, make sure you're choosing a major issue, not a small, incidental one. You must feel certain in your own mind that the insurance company is wrong. If you aren't convinced, you'll never stick to the fight. Winning against a deep-pocketed insurance company takes time, patience, and the confidence to know you are in the right.

And, be warned! If you successfully fight a denial, your victory will only apply to the specific item you're fighting for. If you oppose a claim denial for any other medication or procedure, you'll need to renew the battle. The only advantage next time around is that you'll have learned the ropes for getting the response you want from the insurance company. So if you've made up your mind to fight, go ahead and fight. Become a bulldog!

WORKSHEET - STEPS FOR CONTESTING AN INSURANCE DENIAL

Keep in mind that I am not a lawyer—just a fiercely determined former caregiver. But as a regular claimant up against the insurance system, these are the steps I took to gain a successful decision from our insurance company.

- Contact your insurance agent to find out what's going on. Does he or she need a letter from the doctor before they'll pay for something? Do you need to provide them with information they don't have?

- Consult your state's insurance department to be clear about your rights. Can they help you? Does your state have laws to help protect the policyholder?

- Promptly follow any directions you receive. You may need to take extra steps to retrieve pertinent information, such as doctor reports kept in your record box, etc.

- Hire a lawyer if you don't already have one and communicate with the insurance company only through your attorney.

- Request that the insurance company conduct an outside review of the claim.

- If the final determination is a denial, research the doctor who did the review. Was the correct type of doctor used in evaluating the patient's need?

- Through your lawyer, request a second outside review if something about the first one was incorrect.

- Meanwhile, stay in touch with the state insurance department. Are they able to research the disease for standard of care for the illness, and will they send a letter to the insurance company with a recommendation?

  ○ Standard of care is the treatment being used at the present time in major hospitals for people with the same condition.

- If the second outside review results in a denial, arrange for another outside review you will pay for yourself.

  ○ By this point, you need to be certain you are in the right.

- The insurance company may not give in until they have checked further with the patient's specialist doctor(s) or made other inquiries.

- Remember, all communication must go through your attorney. The insurance company will notify your attorney of their decision.

- If the insurance company agrees to coverage, you win. Being a bulldog has paid off.

- If the company still denies coverage, review with your lawyer the options that remain open to you. Listen to the attorney's advice.

- Research the standard of care for similar cases treated at major hospitals throughout the country. You may be able to sue the insurance company for failing to provide a standard of care.

Fighting an insurance denial isn't easy, and you're already weary as a caregiver. It requires fortitude to continue the fight. Our insurance company took eight months before agreeing to pay Larry's claim. In the meantime, we needed to cover the costs ourselves.

But don't give up. Just because insurance is big business doesn't mean you have no chance to win. Remember, only a small percentage of claimants who are denied fight. That means you aren't going to be hindered by claims from the majority who accept a denial, upping your odds of winning. The bulldogs have the best shot. Will you be one of them?

TWENTY-SEVEN

Remember

Maybe you'll be the caregiver of someone who recovers and goes on to live a full life. Give thanks where it is due and enjoy it. None of us knows how this journey will end.

We also can't say how we're going to manage our circumstances when things don't go well. But we do have control over how we respond if and when they don't. We can assume a key role in easing the pain for our loved one as he or she prepares to pass from this life.

We can also learn about the physical signs of a person's body beginning to transition from life to death. I'm not qualified to explain what happens during the dying process, though your doctor or another professional can provide this information if you desire it. Your local hospice may also have a booklet to explain the physical signs of approaching death in layman's terms.

Nothing is forever. The situation you're facing now isn't either. Something will happen to change things. Neither you nor your loved one asked for this illness or accident. It's not going to magically get better. Some days when you're feeling frazzled, step back and remember you are doing something sacred for another person. Even though you aren't where you want to be, you'll discover a level of strength you didn't realize you possessed. When the day is over and you lay down exhausted but unable to sleep, remind yourself that you're taking on a duty not everyone is capable of fulfilling. Your priority is to help your loved one, and while doing that, you've learned a lot about yourself.

It takes more than one tactic and more than yourself to survive caregiving for your loved one. Through a combination of a positive attitude, hope, faith, lots of help, and medical science, you can survive. When Larry slipped away after a short stay in hospice, my head understood, but my heart was not ready to let him go. Had I done everything right?

No. But I did the best that I could.

As Nora Ephron once said, "*Above all, be the heroine of your life, not the victim.*"

You can do this! I did it, so I know you can too.

TWENTY-EIGHT

Activities For Stress Relief

There is a connection between our hands and mind that can help get you through the stress of caregiving. Those interminable times of waiting beside a bed or for test results, doctor's phone calls, or prescription refills are all opportunities for you to distract your mind. Yes, cell phones do provide some of that distraction, but even they begin to bore after a while.

As a form of self-care, making art offers the calming and grounding benefits of meditation. Even a few minutes of working on a creative project can reduce stress. Instead of focusing on your problems, your mind focuses on the project at hand. By changing the direction of your thoughts, art activities lower your stress level and decrease your feelings of isolation. You stay healthier.

You don't need a background in art in order to enjoy it. You don't even need to be artistic. However, the more engaged you are, the more inspired you become. After all, the creative muscle is like other muscles. The more you use it, the stronger it becomes.

In the midst of caregiving for Larry, with a canvas bag and a bit of planning, I carried a project to work on whenever we left the house. I was always grateful to have it on hand.

Let's get started. What would you like to create?

TWENTY-NINE

Written Journals

When I needed a place to write down everything I was processing as a caregiver, I turned to my journal. What I love about written journals is that they are private, and they can be as plain or as fancy as you wish. There are no rules! All you need is a notebook and a pen.

Extra things to add include stickers, colored pens, markers, a glue stick, and anything you might want to paste into the book.

My journal of choice is those books called "composition books." These books come with various colored covers. They are inexpensive and they're all the same size, making them easier for storage. These journals are also sturdy and attractive; you can throw them in a big purse or a bag to pull out while you're sitting in a doctor's office or picking up an order for delivery. You can write while you wait.

But like any new habit, it can take some time to get used to writing in a journal, especially if it requires reliving a hard day or seeing your emotions processed on the page. If beginning a journal is difficult for you, start by labeling the front of the book with the start date so that when your journal is full, you can add the end date to the front cover. You've just made a commitment to yourself.

To keep yourself from freaking out when you pick up a pen and turn to that first page, write these items across the top line:

- The day of the week, followed by the date.
- Beside the date, draw a half-inch-square "mood box." Use a color code to correspond to your emotions. For example, use a simple system of five colors like black (depressed), blue (sad), purple (pleasant), pink (happy), and red (excited). Whenever you write in the journal, use colored pencils or felt markers to fill in the box indicating your overall mood. Be sure you know what each color means or your code will have no value.

Now that you've gotten past your aversion to writing in a journal, you've started to build a record of your moods. This can be a helpful way to remind you of the ups and downs of a caregiver's journey—and a chance to congratulate yourself for getting through the hard days. Use your journal not just to record your feelings and experiences, but to help you see the big picture:

- How many days did you color your mood box in the mid-color zone? How many days were in the top and how many at the bottom?

- If, after several days, you see a consistent pattern of black or blue boxes, it may be time for you to seek help from a doctor.

If you've only been recording mood boxes so far, how will you start your actual writing? If journal writing is new to you, don't worry about whether it's good or bad. These entries are for you, not for the whole world to see. The point of this journal is to help you sort out your emotions and to keep a record of what's happening.

You might start with one of these questions:

- How do you feel today?

- What happened today to influence how you feel?

After that first entry, keep adding writings each day about the memories you want to keep, things that your loved one said, some place that you or the two of you went, and what you are noticing about the life of a caregiver.

Sometimes, I'd describe places we went or things we talked about. Later, my journals gave me a chance to look back at things I'd have forgotten otherwise.

Don't worry if what you write one day is contradicted by the way you feel on another day. That's part of being human.

A journal is also a good place for lists of all kinds, particularly lists of what you might want to do with your loved one:

- A "someday" list

- A "do tomorrow" list

- A favorite foods list

- A dreams list

- A menus for the week list

If you've had a difficult day or discovered a new problem to solve, write down your challenges, along with some possible solutions. It's often easier to see a solution after you've written down the problem. Write about emotions: resentment, anger, or sadness. Writing releases a lot of the unhappiness you feel. Write about something good, joyous, or happy that has occurred. Acknowledging what you're grateful for can revive your energy for tackling the hard stuff.

Here are some situations you might want to write about:

- How did you feel when you and your loved one left the last doctor appointment?

- If you fixed dinner and your loved one couldn't eat it, how did you feel?

- What did you feel when you were all ready to leave for an appointment and had gotten your loved one into his coat and gloves and he suddenly had to pee?

- Talk about what it felt like to have a recent adventure with your loved one.

If you're struggling to think of a topic to write about, try one of these journal prompts:

- My favorite time of day is . . .

- No one knows this, but I'd love to . . .

- If I could do anything I want, I'd . . .

- My saddest day was . . .

- I'd be so proud if . . .

- I'm happy when . . .

- The best thing about being me is . . .

- Right now, I could use . . .

- My greatest fear is . . .

- The thing I want most is . . .

- Yesterday was the best day, because we . . .

- If I was an animal, I'd be a . . .

Find things that interest you and add them to your journal pages—newspaper or magazine headlines, colors or doodles around the edges. A sticker here and there won't hurt. In my journal, I draw a large B on the margin, circle it, and color it pink to indicate that there's an anecdote about Barney Welsh corgi on the page. Later, if I'm looking for writings featuring my beloved pet, I don't need to read everything. I look for the appropriate marker.

This is your book. Make it look like you. Show who you are during this time. The entries you've made are a reflection of your growth.

Congratulations for taking this step towards lessening your stress.

THIRTY

Art Journals

Art journals are a step beyond written journals confined to the written word. With an art journal, you feature inspiring visuals alongside the words. Sometimes the resulting picture is complete with no words at all. I love this form of expression that's open to virtually anyone. No art training is necessary, and you don't even need to feel creative when you indulge.

Like written journals, this one can either be private or you can share it with others. There are several books about making an art journal, but figuring out the basics is simple. If you find art journaling engaging, feel free to experiment any way you wish.

My first art journal was little more than a written journal with a few colored-in doodles to add more interest to the pages. Somewhere around page six, I daubed the background of the paper with a sponge and a mixture of brown, cream, and orange acrylic paint. I found a picture in a magazine of four older women dressed to go out to dinner. I carefully snipped around the image of each woman and glued them one by one onto the page. I cut out "talk bubbles" from plain white paper and wrote what each woman would be saying about aging. Pasting one bubble above each woman's head, I allowed them to "hold a conversation." Flipping through the magazine once more, I saw a perfect quote on gold-colored paper. I cut it out and pasted it in, giving the page a great message.

The rest of the world might be in chaos, but one character almost demanded dark chocolate be eaten on a continuous basis.

As I grew braver, I began to add bits of fabric, ribbon borders, cut-outs, and a few poorly drawn illustrations to each page, which I tended to cover in my own journal writing. By the time I'd filled all the pages in the first book, my imagination had awoken and I started the second journal while Larry was sick.

While I worked on the pages in this book, my thoughts focused on what might look good on each page. The stress of our situation and Larry's horrible illness receded to the back of my mind, giving me some much-needed relief from constant worry and fear.

Book Two turned out to be much more colorful than the first journal, because I learned something you will already know from reading this section. If the background of the page was already colored, I only needed to add a few pictures or a scrap of fabric, some ribbon, and a bit of journaling. Gradually, the pages began to absorb some of my angst, leaving me with a history of the two-and-a-half years of Larry's illness.

There are no rules in art journaling. You can design the pages any way you wish. Once you've taken this up, you'll develop your own style and favorite materials. That makes sense—your journal should be a reflection of you.

You'll be able to find the following basic art supplies at a craft store or wherever craft supplies are sold:

- A nine-by-eleven-inch or ten-by-ten-inch (approximately) album or memory book with card-stock or heavier weighted pages

- Watercolor or acrylic paint in small bottles (acrylic can be thinned with water to give it a water-color look or used full strength for darker areas)

- A one- or one-and-a-half-inch foam paint brush

- A black gel pen for writing

- A black fine-tipped marker

- A white gel pen

- Magazines

- Scissors

- A glue stick (I use UHU, but other good brands are available)

- Wax paper

- Optional supplies: tissue paper, stickers, ticket stubs, buttons, glitter, bits of fabric, ribbon, lace, scrapbook paper, tape, rubber stamps, doilies, and any other materials you wish. The sky is the limit.

To begin:

1. Paint the background on both sides of about ten pages. Use the same color or different colors for the pages. Place wax paper between the pages so they don't touch each other as they dry.

2. While the paint is drying, think about what you want the page to show. Flip through your magazines for ideas. Clip out a picture.

    a. Example: *Here's a picture of a dog. Look at his cute face. If I cut it out, it could be the centerpiece of the page.*

    b. If your first picture is large, you might not need any others. If your picture is small, look for more pictures to go with the dog and to tell a story. *This little dog looks like he needs a friend. I'll cut one out too.*

3. Continue to search for pictures. Three might be a good number.

4. Arrange and rearrange the pictures on one of your now dry background pages. (It doesn't have to be the first page.)

5. When you like the arrangement, glue the pictures in place using your glue stick.

6. Do you want words on the page? Maybe you want to write about the dog you had as a child or the dog you saw riding down the street in a baby buggy. Use your black marker or pen to write on the page or cut words from the magazine to make a sentence or thought. Glue them in place when you find an arrangement you like.

7. Done! Well, maybe—but there's something not quite finished yet.

8. Perhaps ribbon streamers tied through a hole punched on the side of the page would look good. A fabric heart? Some doodles with black or white pen? What about a border cut from scrapbook paper. Now, daub some glitter here and there. Maybe an odd (one, three, five) number of dots added in clusters with your black or white pen. If you put them in random places, they will fill empty spaces.

9. Survey your work. How does the page look? Feel good about yourself because you've finished the first page in your art journal. The more work you do, the more you'll relax, which only increases the fun.

Sometimes it's easier to start a page with a prompt to get your mind working. Don't overthink an idea, just go with it. This is just for you. It's not meant to be a masterpiece.

- Today I feel like a bird ready to fly to . . .

- I'm angry. What color would that feel like?

- If I were a spy, I'd search for a woman wearing a . . .

- I'd like to be a circus . . .

- What will I pull out of my treasure box?

- Who am I?

- Coffee thoughts

- Tears of sorrow

- Weary, I'm so weary . . .

- At the zoo, I saw . . .

- Sometimes it hurts being left out of things, so I . . .

- Into each life some rain will fall . . .

- The flowers in my garden are . . .

- I'd like to live in a house with . . .

- Draw the outline of the houses on your block or your own house. What could go inside it?

- My favorite color is . . .

- Often quotes will inspire a page. Search for some favorites online.

Poems and simple journal writing are nice additions to any page with a simple ribbon border or a fake flower glued to the corner of the page.

Here's another idea. What about a page to commemorate your anniversary, birthday, or a party? A headline in a magazine or a funny picture might inspire a page. Play with what you find.

At some point, your journal cover needs decorating. It's your book. It only needs to be as fancy as you want it to be. My first one simply said, "Journal #1, Enter At Your Own Risk" written in white pen on a black cover.

As much as I hate to admit it, I have several art journals that aren't finished, but I intend to keep filling the pages of each book. One of the easiest is a color journal with each page dedicated to one color. After doing the colors of the rainbow, I began pages with two colors and even three. It's fun to find pictures and ephemera of a particular color.

Other unfinished journals in my collection include one on Paper Girls, Books I Love, Who Said That?, and one called "All the World's a Stage and All the Men and Women are Players." (Shakespeare)

Even working in the journal for fifteen minutes a day will help you. Have fun and let go of the stress of your life when you can.

I dare you!

THIRTY-ONE

Gratitude Journals

As anyone who's watched a loved one receive a sudden diagnosis knows, your life and future can change in the blink of an eye, and you must decide how you're going to deal with it. Shock may insulate you for the immediate hours or days, but eventually you'll need to figure out how to live with what you've been given. That's when being grateful for what you have is important. It reminds you of all the good things in your life and gives you the strength and energy to keep going.

Larry was fragile and extremely sick when the doctor asked me to move him into a suitable skilled nursing facility (SNF). Although the doctor doubted Larry would survive, after seven weeks, he was able to walk out of the facility.

During the time Larry was in the SNF, I spent long hours by his bedside. Soothing music played while I watched him sleep. Taking a break one day, I went to a craft store to buy supplies for a gratitude journal.

You'll notice this simple project uses many of the same supplies as an art journal. You can also look for these at a craft or discount store:

- A small-sized journal with fifteen or sixteen cardstock pages and a printed cover
- One set of plain black alphabet stickers
- One set of small bubble alphabet stickers or other fancy alphabet stickers that catch your eye
- A glue stick
- Scissors
- A black gel pen
- Two or three pieces of scrapbook paper (optional)
- Several magazines

Now you're ready to make your gratitude journal:

1. My journal was covered with bright paper, but if you can't find one with a pretty pattern, pick up a couple of sheets of scrapbook paper. Cut two rectangular pieces of paper to match the size of the front and back covers. Glue one of the cut sheets to the front and one to the back. Make sure to firmly paste down the edges.

2. What would you like to call your gratitude book? It can be anything that makes you feel good. Mine became, "Heart Flutters Bring Joy." Use the set of plain black alphabet stickers to write the title on the front cover of the book. Add a picture if you wish.

3. Turn to the first page, which will become the title page. Write a quote, a short poem, or a message to explain the purpose of the book. Sign it and add the year you created the journal.

4. Your book will appear more interesting if you paste a border along the loose side of each page. Find magazine pictures of flowers or jewelry for a fun look running down the edges. Layer objects on top of thin, one-color paper strips. Look for geometric, plaid, or paisley patterns to clip from the magazine for borders about half-an-inch wide. Scrapbook paper and doodles work too.

5. Go through the book and place one letter (bubble or fancy ones) onto the front and one onto the back of each page. If your book has fifteen pages, you'll have room for one letter on each sheet. (My book didn't have enough pages, so I doubled up some of the less frequently used letters.) Place one alphabet letter anywhere along the upper part of each page, leaving room for the things you'll use to embellish each one.

6. Now comes the fun part: finding magazine images of things you love and are grateful to have in your life. Clip them out and glue the pictures randomly on the correct alphabet page. Words cut from publications work great if you scatter them among the photos. Add some handwritten words or illustrations for items you can't find in your magazines. If you use your imagination, you'll be able to add images from all five senses. How about "baking bread" for the letter B? If you can't find a picture of bread, cut out the word from your magazines or, better yet, draw your own version of "baking bread."

7. Continue to add to your book of blessings as time goes by. Add lace, ribbons, stickers, or anything you want to make it special.

I hope your gratitude journal will become one of your joy-makers.

THIRTY-TWO

Making Hearts

When I was caring for Larry, he suffered from constant headaches, which his doctor did not attribute to the brain tumor. A headache specialist attempted to reduce the pain by using all kinds of painkillers and even Botox shots. Nothing worked until she suggested the cause might be due to an injury earlier in his life. She recommended physical therapy.

When Larry was nineteen, he'd worked on a road crew pouring concrete. One day the box from a dump truck flew down toward him. He moved his head just in time to keep from losing it. He suffered from severe whiplash.

Fifty years later, here we were, hoping we'd discover the cause of the pain. Four days a week, we traveled from The Flying Saucer Campground in Englewood across Denver to Aurora. Larry gradually found relief from the intensive therapy since a lot of it focused on his neck. Each hour-long session gave me time to work on a project while I waited for him. My idea of sewing small hearts wasn't anything new, but they kept my hands busy and, since the hearts were small and delicate, my mind didn't wander.

I learned that there were several ways to use the hearts, and would argue that a project like this is something anyone can do and enjoy. They look cute draped along a wall or the top of a window like a valance. They could hang on a small tree found at a craft store. The tree could be a small Christmas tree, a metal tree with arms extending outward, a branch stuck in a can, or anything else you'd want to use. Your hearts might be made with a theme in mind like the Fourth of July. You might give visitors a handmade heart when they leave after seeing you and your loved one. Use them for a matching game: find the two hearts with a brown stripe, etc.

You can look for other creative ideas on Pinterest or a similar site. Let your thoughts focus on this simple task for a short time. Enjoy feeling capable without any added responsibility.

Here are a few materials to consider. These simple supplies fit in a tote bag:

- Two pieces of white paper
- A pencil

- Scissors
- Pinking shears (optional)
- Scraps of different-colored cotton fabrics (as many as you want)
- Loose cotton stuffing or cotton balls
- A needle
- White and black thread
- Embroidery thread (optional, but it offers more color options)
- A few straight pins
- Ribbon, if the hearts are going to be hung or draped on a wall
- Embellishments, such as lace, ribbon, small buttons (optional)
- Fabric glue

1. Fold one sheet of paper in half like a hot dog.

2. Using your pencil, draw half a heart along the fold. How large do you want it?

3. Cut the heart out, open it, and you will have a pattern for your first heart.

4. Make several more heart patterns, each of a different size.

5. Select the fabrics you wish to use.

6. Fold the cloth in half and pin a pattern onto it. This makes a front and a back.

7. Cut around your heart patterns using a pair of pinking shears or regular fabric scissors until you have a dozen or so pairs.

8. Pin each pair of hearts together with their right sides facing out.

9. Sew the heart pairs together using black or white thread or various colors of embroidery thread. Since you're sewing on the outside of the fabric, the stitches will show. Move in from the edge of the fabric by a quarter of an inch. Leave an unsewed area on one side about an inch long to use as an entryway for stuffing.

10. Push your cotton stuffing or cotton balls into the heart. When you feel the heart is plump enough, go back to where you stopped sewing and finish closing the hole.

11. If you want to add embellishments, do that now. Sew or glue them onto the hearts.

12. Add a thread hanger for placing the hearts on a tree. Sew them together at the widest point to drape them on a wall or as a valance.

You can do the same thing with any shape you think up. What about dogs or cats? A string of paper dolls? Your paper patterns don't resemble major works of art? So what? This is your project. Enjoy it. Have fun!

THIRTY-THREE

Happiness Keys

We talk a lot about happiness, and even during this rough period of caring for your loved one, it's important to look for joy and remind yourself of phrases or quotes that inspire a sense of peace. When Larry was sick, I often found myself on a hunt for things that lifted my spirits. One day, I spotted a book in a bookstore by Alexandra Stoddard called *Choosing Happiness*. After reading this book and quickly forgetting much of what I'd read, I thought of something better: a set of "happiness keys." I didn't have to memorize happy thoughts; I could just flip through these keys whenever I needed an uplift.

I realized that happiness keys would make excellent gifts for anyone else needing encouragement.

To make your own keys, here's what you'll need:

- Scrapbook paper (cardstock weight). Look for simple patterns and solid colored paper. You can use each page more than once for your set of keys

- A "key-shaped" stencil

- A pencil

- Scissors

- A black gel pen

- A white gel pin

- A hole punch

- A key ring (mine is a metal one from Walmart)

- Positive phrases (collected from wherever you can find them)

- Alphabet stamps (optional)

- A stamp pad (optional)

- Stickers (optional)

Now, you're ready to get started:

1. Place the key stencil on the scrapbook paper and use it to trace as many paper keys as you want. You might start with twenty and add more if you feel like it.

2. Cut them out.

3. Punch a hole at the top of each key.

4. Write your name and date on the first key of the bunch. For example: "Carol's Happiness Keys." Below that, mark down the year you made the keys.

5. Using your black pen on light-colored paper and your white pen on dark paper, write one phrase on each key. Spread the words out so they have a pleasing appearance. If you're using alphabet stamps, do the same thing.

6. Add stickers, drawings, or other small items for embellishment if you'd like.

7. Thread the keys onto the key ring.

Choose from these phrases or make up your own:

Kindness, kindness, kindness!	Smiles are free
Be tolerant	Be generous to others
Look for the good	Read good books
Be thankful	Stay curious
Trust yourself	Meditate often
Stay organized	Be yourself
Patience pays off	Never, never give up
Stay positive	Love life
Love with all your heart	Encourage others
Be genuine	Laugh loudly
Think positive thoughts	Enjoy nature
Stay loyal	Live in the moment
Colors are magic	Treat others well
Play like a child	Keep a sense of humor
Dream big	Stay hopeful
Do for others	Choose carefully
Let your imagination inspire you	Cheer yourself with music
Enjoy being creative	Enjoying your pets
Be humble	Accept what you can't change
Forgive others	Know yourself

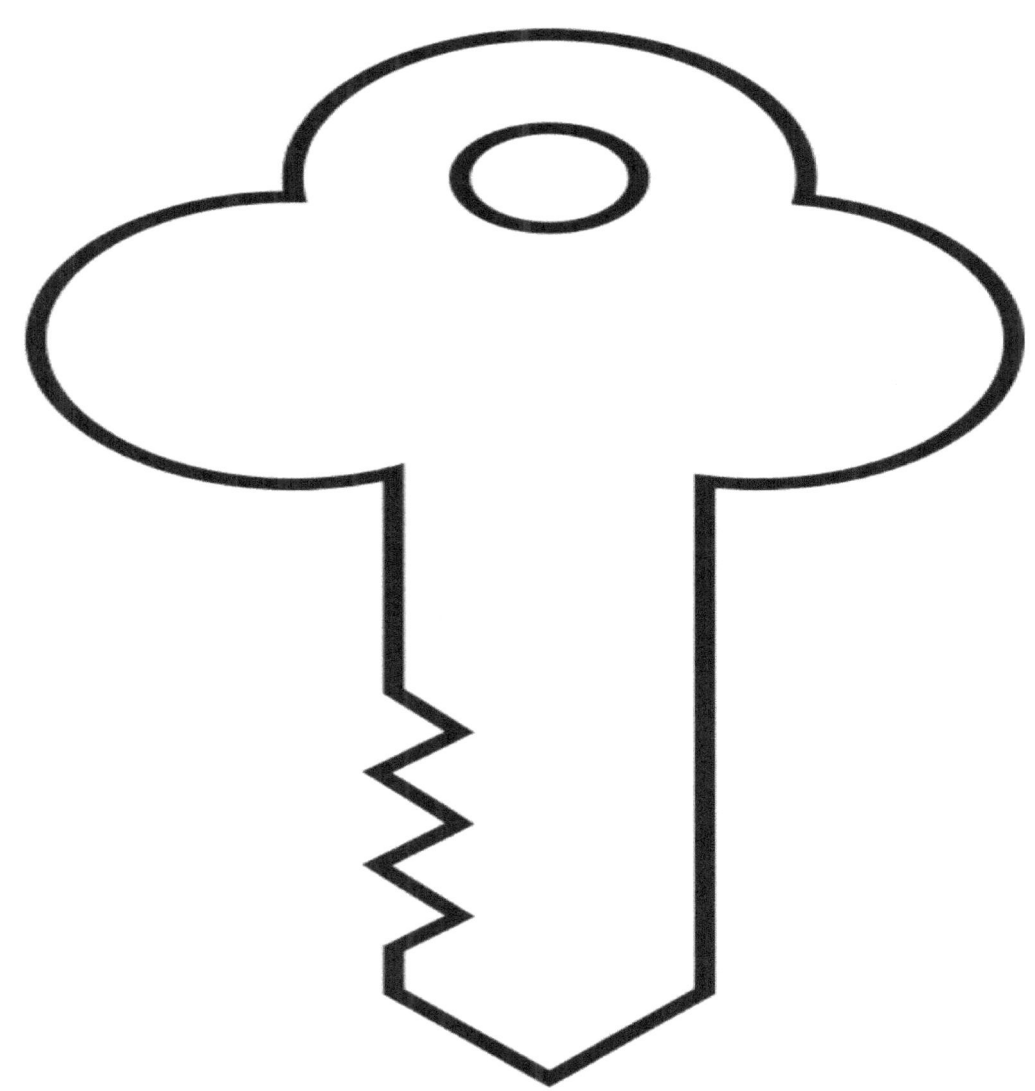

THIRTY-FOUR

Conclusion

By now you've had time to absorb the basics of your new role as a caregiver. The shock is past, and I hope you've made time to try an art activity or two. Because these projects are designed to keep you more emotionally stable, there is no room for guilty feelings. This is for your mental health.

If writing in your journal is the most you can manage at this time, that's okay. You have an outlet for part of the frustration and anxiety you face. To bring some fun into it, next time try a pen with a different color ink. Add some doodles or a few stickers that make you smile. Add a little sunshine to your writing journal.

Try another project. You aren't required to work on them each day. Some days don't leave you with time or energy. Look forward with anticipation to the next opportunity for you to continue letting yourself enjoy your time even if it's for only fifteen minutes.

Although not mentioned as a project in this book, watercolor painting is a delicious way to lessen the seriousness of your situation for a short time. One day, I got out paper and watercolor paints for my husband. Since he was a trucker kind of guy, he had a great time painting a truck. We talked and laughed as he tried his hand at something he hadn't attempted since childhood.

Your situation will change. Everything does. You are doing a great job of keeping it all together. With some art projects to distract you from worries about the future, you'll feel more alive. So, give yourself some minutes of happiness.

About the Author

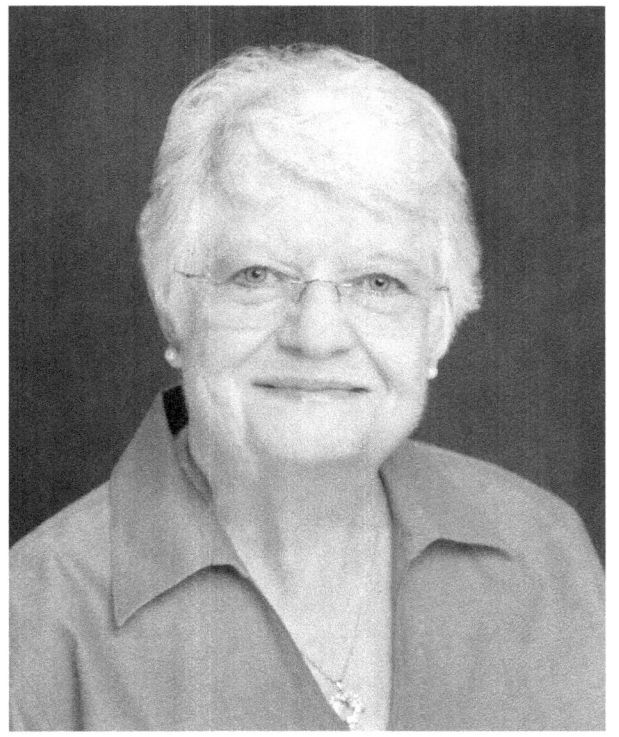

Carol Chapman starts her day with two cups of coffee and the morning quietness she craves. When she isn't writing, Carol loves reading, movies (especially when they include popcorn), lunching with friends, volunteering, and dark, rich chocolate anytime, anywhere.

Stories about ordinary women who discover their strengths are her favorites, ranging from memoir to light mysteries to historical fiction. Books spill out of all corners of her home.

Carol lives with her favorite guy, Barney Pembroke Welsh Corgi Chapman, in her native state of Wyoming.

Carol's memoir, *Finding the Good: A Journey through Love, Loss, and Living* was published in 2024.

Photo by Audie Jeans Photography

Twice a month, you can enjoy reading Carol's blog, Engaging While Aging, centered around finding the good in everyday life. Meet Barney Welsh Corgi and learn about some curiosities of today and yesterday.

https://carolchapmanwrites.com.

www.ingramcontent.com/pod-product-compliance
Lightning Source LLC
Chambersburg PA
CBHW081719120626

46550CB00010B/3172